MY HEART MADE NEW

Bill Yeomans

Books by Bill Yeomans
Book 1 <u>Power Versus</u> - To Strengthen Your Walk
Book 2 <u>The Face of God</u> – Reflected in Nature
Book 3 <u>Christ Centered Marriages</u> – Your Marriage Matters
Book 4 <u>Christ Centered Finances</u> – Your Money Matters
Book 5 <u>Christ Centered Families</u> – Your Kids Matter
Book 6 <u>Bill I AM – An Autobiography</u>
Book 7 <u>My Heart Made New</u>
SOON TO BE RELEASED:
Book 8 <u>The Spirit of God</u>
Book 9 <u>America Needs God</u>
Book 10 <u>Tough Men for Tough Times</u>

CONTENTS

DISCLAIMER

Nothing in this book should be construed to offer medical advice. All opinions and recommendations offered in this book are taken from, and as a result of, the personal experience and observations of the author. The information contained in this book is in no way intended to offer medical or psychological advice or solutions. All medical decisions and choices should be made only at the advice of, and under consultation with, a medical professional.

ABOUT THE AUTHOR

B ill Yeomans is a Heart Survivor! He has suffered and survived seven (7) Heart Attacks. Each one was the result of him making uninformed and under-informed lifestyle choices. He has been an active person all of his life. Bill has led teenagers on cross-country hikes as well as canoe trips in the High Sierra. Bill and his wife Marelene, have raised six children. They have been blessed with ten grandchildren. They have been married for 54 years and counting. During these years, Bill has served as Pastor to seven churches. He has built a two-story house and barn from the ground up. He has served his country as a U S Naval Officer, making two cruises in the South China Sea as division officer aboard the aircraft carrier, USS Ranger, CVA-61 during the Vietnam War. He also served as Assistant Security Officer of the United States Naval War College. Bill has also lived the last twenty years in a state of denial. From the time of his very first heart attack, he has simply accepted his condition as a natural part of life. Consequently, he has done little to change his life style. He has endured heart vessel angioplasty, arterial stents, and finally a triple bypass surgery. Still, his lifestyle changed very little.

During Heart Attack number six, Bill was told by his surgeon that no further physical intervention was possible. All of the previously grafted vessels were totally occluded (blocked) with the exception of <u>one single vessel supplying blood to keep the heart muscle alive</u>! Basically, he was told to go home and put his affairs in order.

Six months later along came Attack Number Seven! This time the medical team spent two weeks attempting to stabilize Bill in order to keep him alive. During this time Pastor Bill reflected deeply as to why God had seen fit to allow him to live. Bill knew that for many years he had desired to write a book, but had always put it off for a later time. He, like many of you, was a "<u>master of procrastination</u>"! After attack number seven, he dared to make a bargain with God! Pastor Bill made a promise to God that for every day God allowed him to live, Bill Yeomans would write and work on his first book. He further promised that it would be a book to help others and to honor God. Four months later his first book was completed and published under the title "<u>Power Versus to Strengthen Your Walk</u>". At the time of this writing, God has granted Pastor Bill in excess of 730 more days! During this "Grace Period" Pastor Bill Yeomans has written and published seven (7) books and has several more in progress. This book is his testimony of how this has become possible!

This is only part of his amazing testimony! "<u>My Heart Made New</u>" is this author's testimony of how he found a whole new style of living. **This is not a book on dieting**!! Instead, it is a personal testimony of how God used some exceptional people to open his eyes and his heart (pun intended) to a whole new way to approach every aspect of living. His story will bless you whether or not you (currently) have any "Heart Issues"!

FORWARD

After my seventh heart attack on July 10, 2015, I was totally resigned to a life which consisted of getting my affairs in order so that my death would be as painless as possible to my wife and family. I had dared to make a bargain with the Lord. I promised that if He would allow me to live even a few more days, I would write a book. I promised to write every single day until this book was accomplished. I further promised this would be a book to honor God and help people. This book, "<u>Power Verses to Strengthen Your Walk</u>" was published four months later on November 16, 2015. Twenty-Four months have passed and I have written and published not one, but six books! God is so merciful! This book is number seven! And it is significantly different from all the others!

This 'Forward' is being written on December 30, 2016, which just happens to be my 79th birthday! In the last six months, I have found a totally new approach to living. Instead of waiting to die, I am now looking forward toward many more years of excited living for Christ!

This book, "<u>My Heart Made New</u>" is my personal testimony about how God has intervened in my life and totally changed my attitude toward living! My prayer is that God will use this book to help you gain victory in whatever struggles you might be going through now or in the future.

I am so totally committed to sharing my story, that I am asking you to share it with everyone you know and care deeply about. In fact, I am offering to do something that may sound crazy...... If, after reading this book, you wish to share a copy with a friend, but you cannot afford to do this, send me an e-mail with the pertinent information and I will send a <u>free copy</u> to your friend. No questions asked! Only one free copy per reader please!

I am also making this book available as an E-Book on the AMAZON – KINDLE platform. The e- book is available to read for free or to purchase for $0.99! A Paperback version is also available on AMAZON.

May God bless you, as you allow Him to change your life for the better!

Bill Yeomans
william.yeomans.fb@gmail.com

GOD RESCUED ME

"GOD RESCUED ME FROM THE GRAVE

AND NOW MY LIFE IS FILLED WITH LIGHT.

YES, GOD OFTEN DOES THESE THINGS FOR
PEOPLE.

HE RESCUES THEM FROM THE GRAVE

SO THEY MAY LIVE IN THE LIGHT OF THE LIVING"
(JOB 33:28-30)

DEDICATION

This book is dedicated to all the friends and family members

who have stood beside me, and my loved ones,

during these many years of attempting

to remain true and faithful to our Lord.

Your acts of love and kindness have

made the difference when times were tough.

Your commitment to God and the reality of His faithfulness

has done much to build my resolve. Thank you for your support

and your love, tempered with a certain amount of

Bill Yeomans

'Tough Love' when you knew I needed it.

I fully expect that you will keep living for Him.

God Bless each one of you!

CHAPTER 1
CONFIDENCE

Confidence is not always a positive quality. I can be confident that I have a problem. I can also be confident that I know one or more solutions to that problem. However, confidence itself is not a solution! Confidence isn't worth anything unless it is followed by positive action. I am confident that more people will die from heart disease in the United States of America than from any other single cause. Why am I this confident? Simply because this fact has been substantiated by a great deal of statistical analysis. This has been backed up by hard scientific facts. Yes, indeed folks, heart disease is number one! Just as I am confident of this fact, I am also confident of the solution! I invite you to pay attention! Here comes the train!

STOP, LOOK AND LISTEN
My son and his family live in the Eastern part of Colorado which forms the beginning of the Great Plains. Through his tiny town pass several freight trains every day. These trains

consist of approximately 100 cars fully loaded with coal heading towards the Gulf states and the eastern seaboard. Many of the Railroad Intersections that cross country roads have no physical barriers or warning lights. The only warning of potential doom is a rather small black and white sign in the shape of an X which says "Railroad Crossing, Stop, Look and Listen!" Sadly, there are several persons killed at such crossings every year in spite of the signs. People are killed simply because they refused to acknowledge and act upon the danger.

Stopping at a railroad crossing is not merely a suggestion. Rather, it is an imperative command! The average weight of a Diesel-Electric locomotive, by itself, can be up to 190 long tons. Add to this the weight of any railcars attached to the engine, and we have a truly formidable force! When placed in motion, this force can become deadly! Any person who would choose to ignore the sign would be considered foolish at the very least!

How does a railroad crossing sign equate with all the beneficial signs for healthy eating? First and foremost, we need to stop the direction in which we are heading. We have to be convinced of the impending disaster if we do not stop. Everyone knows that a moving train can kill you. No one would deny this! The difficulty comes when we try to compare a tiny blood clot with an onrushing locomotive. The two just do not equate, or do they? I'm an old math teacher. At times, I like to look at the laws of probability. I would suggest that the probability of being hit by a freight train is similar to that of being struck by lightning. With the tiniest bit of preventive planning we can reduce these odds even more. Merely following simple suggestions like, "Don't sit under a large tree during a lightning storm". Or "Look both ways and listen before crossing the railroad intersection". No person, no matter how foolish, should disregard such simple suggestions to stay alive.

There is a killer that is far deadlier than an oncoming train or a lightning bolt. A tiny blood clot or a loose chunk of plaque can kill you just as fast and leave you just as dead! It can also cause you a great deal of pain while you are in the process of dying. And, like the onrushing train, or the lightning bolt, we seldom see it coming! Why? Because many of us are living in a constant state of denial. We live with the mistaken belief that something this terrifying can never happen to us. Many of us will continue to live in this state of denial until it is too late. Sadly, most of us do not worry or concern ourselves about the possibility of developing blood clots or plaque within our arteries! These are the hidden killers. The ones lying in ambush. Ready to strike at a moment's notice! These are the silent killers. Therefore, they are easy to deny. They can be readily ignored. That is, until they strike a deadly blow! <u>You might consider me an expert since I have the dubious distinction of having survived seven full-blown heart attacks!</u> Have I got your attention yet? Or are you still in some kind of a deep state of denial?

This book is my personal testimony that it is possible to reverse coronary heart disease without adding one single pill to your dietary regimen. I am living, breathing proof of this assertion! I have nothing to gain monetarily. Any profit I may gain from this book will be given away to worthwhile charities for the prevention and treatment of heart disease. I am a Christian author. I have discovered a simple way to save lives. I would be a hypocrite if I did not share this with anyone willing to listen.

Here is a proven fact: <u>Heart Disease is the number one killer of both men and women in the industrialized world.</u> Not cancer! Cancer is the number two cause. Not accidents! Accidents that occur in the medical-care field are the third greatest cause of death. Strokes are the number four cause of death. News Flash! <u>Heart Disease is number one</u>! Here is a second newsflash! Medical records indicate that a full 50% of all heart attack victims died as a result of their first heart attack! Here comes the Good News: **Death by heart disease is preventable!** It is most often caused by a simple case of <u>ignorance</u> and <u>denial</u> of the facts! If I sound like a preacher at this point, it is because I am a preacher! In fact, I have been a preacher for over 50 years! However, this book is not a series of sermons, but a personal testimony. It is about a truth that has been known for some time. Simply stated, we are what we eat! And what we eat determines how we will then live! Or how we will die.

Here is my story.

CHAPTER 2

AN AMAZING DISCOVERY

I t might be said that what follows is the result of an ac-
cident or a matter of chance. Personally, I do not believe
in anything happening by mere chance. I believe God has
a plan for each of us. I believe he has a purpose for you
and for me. I believe that my purpose right now is to share
with you a simple discovery that has changed my life for the
better. It all began when I 'stumbled' upon a book entitled
"The China Study". This is a well-documented study by a
renowned nutritionist who undertook an exhaustive study
involving 60 out of 62 provinces in the country of China.
This was a study of the eating habits of farmers and peas-
ants in the rural areas of China. This was done over a period of 12 years. One of the most startling discoveries was
that the so-called diseases of the industrialized world were
practically nonexistent among the rural people of China.
Both heart disease and diabetes were practically unheard
of! Obesity and high blood pressure were also conditions
that were virtually unknown to this population. What was

the common denominator? What made these people so different? Putting it simply; everything that was discovered was directly related their diet. It was what they ate that made the difference! It was what they refrained from eating that made the difference. It was the volume of certain foods they ate that made the difference. It was how their bodies reacted to what they ate that made the difference. This was so simple it was actually profound!

I am a sceptic by nature. I started my professional career as a Naval Officer and subsequently as an eighth-grade science teacher. I do not accept opinions or assumptions as fact. I have always demanded to see the proof of any idea or hypothesis. As I started to read this book, 'The China Study', my skepticism kicked into overdrive! I was determined to find the flaws in what was being presented as fact. If this was true, why had no one discovered it before? Why was this so called 'miracle' only now being uncovered? I confess that I had many questions with very few answers. But this information was so intriguing that I determined to dig in and find out some answers for myself. Was it, in fact, possible to prevent such diseases as Congestive Heart Disease and Coronary Artery Disease along with Type Two Diabetes simply by changing what one puts in his or her mouth? Furthermore, was it possible to reverse these diseases through diet alone or by a combination of diet and exercise? I decided to make it my top priority to dig in and find out the truth. What was the China Study all about? What were the credentials of these authors? What were the parameters and controls associated with the study? And most importantly, who was the funding source behind the study?

I needed to discover the answers to, Who? What? Why? and How?

The China Study was the first and by far the most exhaustive and complete study of the eating habits of a large and diverse population ever attempted. Today, more than twenty years later, it is still considered to be the 'Gold Standard' of all such studies.

The credentials of the father-son authors are impeccable! Both men are well known and widely respected in their respective fields. In the past few years, several other books have been written by prominent heart specialists confirming these findings. In the back of this book you will find an index crediting some of the books that have meant the most to me in my personal walk. In the past few months I have endeavored to compile a list of some of the more believable and well-known authors who are continuing to advance the study of healthy living without the benefit of animal protein and animal fat. Some of these are listed in the back of this book under "<u>Further Resources For Your Consideration</u>"

I have absolutely no personal or financial interest in any of these books. They are included in the index for the sole purpose of helping you verify what I'm attempting to share. I am certain there are others that are equally informative, which I have yet to discover.

CHAPTER 3

EATING OURSELVES TO DEATH

In essence, the industrialized world is eating itself to death! Our newly found affluence over the past 50 years has developed into refining and modifying our eating habits and food sources into something far removed from their natural state. Why in the world would we do such a thing? The obvious answer lies in the fact that we have evolved into people who are constantly on the go. In the United States, we only need to look at the last 100 years of our history in order to understand why this has taken place. We have changed from a society that primarily lived at home and worked very close to home. Travel was a difficult situation at best. For thousands of years man walked where he wanted to go. Travel was vastly improved with the ability to domesticate the horse. Now man could travel 20 to 30 miles in one day. When we learned how to harness steam power we could travel by train and steam powered ships great distances in relatively short periods of time. World War II changed our perspective on almost every aspect of our lives. Women were no longer expected to stay at home. With many men gone off to war, there was the need for women to take their places in the factories. It was no longer expected that a women's place was in the home. In fact, just the opposite became true. Women came into their own right as legitimate workers outside of the home. With added income, came higher expectations. Women no longer had time or a desire to stay at home and cook nutritious meals. The food industry was quick to learn that the general populace wanted more fast and easily prepared meal choices. They were quick to respond! This was the beginning of what was to become the fast food frenzy that we know today. Everything from instant rice to frozen dinners became the norm almost overnight. Why peel a potato when you had instant potatoes in the box? No one seemed to care or even realize that what was being gained in expediency was being lost in nutritional value. Even such staples as oatmeal were offered in their "instant variety". This trend literally exploded with the invention of the microwave oven. Now every meal could be an instant meal. Dinner literally became a six-minute voyage from the freezer, to the microwave, to the table! People were too busy to even venture out to the restaurants for a sit-down meal. Almost overnight, 'fast-food, take-out' became a reality!

Many families In the USA find it necessary for both parents to work in order to maintain their desired standard of living. Because of this, it is no longer possible for one parent to spend most of their day in the home. Most wives and mothers are no longer able to spend long hours at home.

They no longer have time to purchase and cook the wholesome meals that were commonplace 50 years ago. In many homes meals are no longer eaten together as a family. For many families, this scenario might look like Mom stopping by after work to grab a pizza at the pizza shop or 'take-out' at a fast food outlet or grabbing some prepared meal to take home to her family. After working all day, she might choose to stop by the grocery store and buy a few frozen dinners to pop in the microwave as soon as she gets home. Needless to say, many of these fast food alternatives do not offer the healthiest food choices. Many of these processed meals no longer have much of the original nutrition found in whole grains, fresh fruits and vegetables. In addition, many of them are loaded down with additives proven to be harmful to our bodies. Saturated fat is just one of these proven killers. This is used for preparing almost all of our dearly loved deep-fried foods. In many industrialized nations, we are literally shortening our lives every time we open our mouths! Fast food has become our 'food of the future'. It has also become our food of the present. Fast food with all of it's shortcuts to nutrition is also killing us at a faster pace than ever before!

CHAPTER 4

UPSIDE – DOWNSIDE

I can think of many reasons not to go on a vegetarian or vegan diet. The concept of a bland taste experience with certain yucky vegetables might top my list.

Collard greens and Kale are two of my least favorite 'Greens'. In my opinion, no child or adult should be forced to eat them! Not when there are so many really delicious green colored veggies out there. Green Vegetables contain many, many, many truly beneficial ingredients. You start with Spinach and Swiss Chard with all their high-powered Iron and Proteins. Next, we could add cruciferous vegetables such as cauliflower, brussels sprouts and cabbage. Add the king of all veggies, broccoli! I can almost hear some of you readers gasping in disgust and maybe even with a bit of horror! Please don't panic! There are many different ways to disguise the flavor of things you do not especially care for. There are ways to make you love the most unlovable veggies you can imagine! There are several excellent vegetarian recipe books on the market today to help get you started and keep you interested and perhaps even excited!

When John Paul Jones was asked by his first Lieutenant <u>if they should keep on fighting</u>, John Paul Jones is quoted as saying, "Don't give up the ship!" Now this answer can be interpreted in two very different ways: "Don't! Give up the ship! This answer would signify he was ready to surrender. However, a simple change in the punctuation would give a totally different answer! "Don't give up the ship!" Means we should keep fighting to the death. So, I ask the question, "Are you ready to make the commitment to change your eating habits for the rest of your life"? Weigh your commitment carefully before you answer. Your positive commitment will not only change your quality of life, but may also add years to your life!

Most decisions in life have both a positive and a negative consequence. The trickiest part of making decisions comes when we need to weigh one side against the other. What will I lose, what will I gain?

THE DOWNSIDE

Let's begin with the argument concerning what I will need to give up. In the early years of my life we did not have much meat on the table for the simple reason that we could not afford it! After graduating from college, I moved up the socio economic ladder and was able to afford more of the so-called luxury items found in the grocery stores. These included such delicacies as ribeye steak, roast beef, pork chops and all sorts of barbecue treats. I quickly developed a taste for this type of food. I was also able to afford butter instead of margarine. In fact, I developed a wonderful taste for butter! My idea of 'eating my veggies' consisted of corn on the cob slathered with butter! Butter on the mashed potatoes. Butter on the outside of the slices of white bread filled with thick slices of cheddar cheese and grilled to perfection. Oh yes, butter was my friend! Gravy was another one of my special friends. Brown gravy, mushroom gravy, white gravy, chicken gravy, pork gravy and beef gravy. I loved almost every kind of gravy. What amazes me today, is that it took so long for my arteries to clog up and present me with my first heart attack!

A roasted 'rib-end' of a pork loin was by far my favorite! This was a succulent delicacy! I thought this was as close to heaven as I ever could get while still on earth. Little did I realize that eating all this animal fat was speeding me along towards my trip to heaven!

As I am describing my previous eating delights, bacon and eggs would have to top the list. This was followed by barbecue Pork Ribs. Another favorite of mine was almost any kind of cheese. Mac and cheese? You bet! All of these things were truly a lot to give up! That was the downside.

THE UPSIDE
The upside to this equation is pure and simple. By choosing to give up all of the foods that were clogging my arteries and setting me up for all of these heart attacks, I gained a new lease on life. Not only have I already lived two years longer than predicted by my doctors, but the quality of my life has vastly improved. To me, this is a "no-brainer"! To me, the decision to eat a vegetarian/vegan diet has allowed me to continue doing the things I love to do with the people I love to be with. In my humble opinion life does not get

much better! Do I miss the old foods? I'd be a liar to tell you "never". Have I made the commitment? Absolutely!

This book is my testimony about the upside of my decision. This is about the upside of my new way of living. This is about how God has allowed me to beat all odds. This is about how God loves me and is honoring my decision to live for Him!

CHAPTER 5

CHOOSING TO COMMIT

LIP SERVICE OR LIFE SERVICE?

When I was a young lad there was a popular song titled "Love and Marriage" The Lyrics went something like this: 'Love and marriage, love and marriage, go together like a horse and carriage. Dad was told by Mother. You can't have one. You can't have one. You can't have one without the other.' Perhaps the popularity of this song lent itself to the concept that marriage was sacred. Back then, marriage was a commitment. Marriage was a sacred promise between two individuals. It was a promise to be kept and fulfilled for better or for worse, for richer or for poorer, in sickness and in health, as long as they both should live. In many areas of the world the concept of marriage commitment has become somewhat of a joke. The word 'commitment' has often been substituted for the term 'convenience'.

This book is about a commitment I have made to restore my body and my soul to a healthier condition. It is not something I take lightly. It is not some fad or spectacular diet. This is a commitment I have made to myself and to my God. This is a commitment I fully intend to keep!

Sadly, I have discovered that when I share this discovery, folks will seldom ask a single question about what happened to change me. More often they respond with a platitude of socially acceptable buzzwords to make themselves and me feel better. Most folks have absolutely no intention of changing their lifestyle, even if it means saving their life. Our modern, indulgent society has become far too complacent. Their new theme song could be "Get it while it's hot, and deny me not".

One dear lady who has struggled with her weight for many years responded to me in the following manner: "Oh I could never do that, I like my meat and potatoes!" Another equally overweight lady responded with a polite smile while stating "This just cannot work for me since I get most all my food at the food bank". Please forgive me if this sounds judgmental! If you find yourself in this category, let me encourage you right here and now. If you truly want to change to a healthier style of eating, God will help you do it! He wants you to feel good. He wants you to feel good about yourself. God wants to help you! Just have the courage to ask Him!

A FACE OR A MOTHER
What do we mean when we categorize any living organism as one who has never had either a face or a mother? First, we need to ask ourselves, "Is this statement inclusive or is it exclusive? Are we attempting to include a certain group or category, or are we trying to exclude certain individuals or groups or categories? In this case, perhaps the most honest answer is, "BOTH"!

The consensus of thought recently being developed in the modern medical community, is that protein derived from plant sources is far more desirable than protein from members of the animal, bird, or fish families. More and more research seems to indicate that <u>the most harmful source of protein for human consumption</u> is found in any type of red meat. This being closely followed by all types of foul such as turkey and chicken. It's been said that "Only a goose will consider eating a goose"! Obviously, I'm not sure who made that statement! The point being, is that geese are filled with too much grease, and are among some of the most 'foul' creatures in the animal kingdom.

Among the creatures that roam the land and inhabit the waters of the world, this leaves the third most harmful source of protein to include fish and other sea creatures. If you are absolutely committed to eating any member of the animal kingdom, I would suggest limiting your intake to creatures of the sea. This protein is by far the least harmful as long as you don't overindulge and become 'done-in' with mercury poisoning.

What does that leave us with? The plant kingdom, naturally! Only plants do not have a face and never have had a mother. Unless, of course, we consider the beautiful face of a Sunflower. However, for the sake of this discussion, we will define a face as having at least one or more of the following features, including a mouth or nose, with eyes to see and ears to hear.

Let's stop right here and mention one of the most popular arguments against a plant-based diet. As my wife once stated, "How in the world are you going to get enough protein?" "Even if you did like tofu, which I know you do not, you would still have to eat some meat and fish in order to have a balanced diet and get enough protein." She continued, " Have you considered that you need to eat fish in order to get enough omega-3?" Needless to say, my wife Marelene, was not in favor of my suggestion that a mostly vegetable and whole-grain diet was going to be healthy for me. In fact, just the opposite is true! The truth of the matter is that it took numerous months and several lab reports before she started to become a believer in what I was attempting to do. It surely is not easy to overcome public opinion when it seems to be championed by the one you love the most! I recognized from the very beginning that she was not going to participate in cooking these 'bland, disgusting meals'! Even today, many months later, I still find myself doing most of my cooking. And that's okay! I have to ask myself, "Why would I ask the one I love to participate in an activity in which she has had severe doubts?" Only some egotistical narcissist would try something like that! If we really love the ones we claim to love, we need to cherish and respect their opinions and their values even more than our own. This makes me the 'happy vegan cook' in my home!

"TRUTH ALERT" <u>It is never right</u> to attempt to force my values on anyone else, **<u>never</u>**! If I quietly live out my system of values, others may see something of value in my life and may ask me to explain. It is at this point that I have been given permission to share my values and life decisions with others. This is true with spiritual values as well as how we find enough protein to sustain a healthy body. I believe you have given me such permission to share by your simple act of purchasing this book!

When committing to any long-term regimen, we need to install some type of a relief valve so that when the pressure gets too great, we don't explode! My self-imposed relief valve is to visit a favorite restaurant and order deep fried calamari steaks. As long as I do this infrequently I don't even feel guilty! Another one of my escape plans is to order one or two bean burritos to go along with my normal diet of veggies. At this point in time I don't even miss the taste of beef or bacon! "Thank you, Jesus!"

So, what's the big deal about eating vegetables? I am a guy who has always loved veggies. I love them almost as much as I love meat and potatoes along with plenty of gravy! Especially that thick greasy gravy! It is simply delicious! Newsflash, it is also deadly! For 77 years of my life I have thoroughly enjoyed eating the American diet. A juicy pork roast with mashed potatoes and lots of gravy is a meal to die for! (Which I almost did!) It's almost as good as a ribeye steak cooked on the barbecue along with a baked potato and lots of butter and sour cream. Topping off a meal like this with Apple Pie à la mode made me feel like I was in heaven! (Little did I know how close I was!) I often made jokes such as "Pie without cheese is like a kiss without a squeeze". I would jokingly say, "I only like two kinds of pie, hot and cold". This would always get a polite laugh from the crowd. Little did they know they were laughing me right into the grave.

Sadly, it is the American diet that has almost killed me seven times! Not only have I endured seven major heart attacks, but my body has also been a distinguished carrier of type II diabetes, high blood pressure, and excessive belly fat. Thankfully, much of the belly fat evaporated about 18 months ago, while the blood pressure is normal and the diabetes is vastly improved!

I'm usually a pretty quick learner, except when it comes to the things I love to eat. Over the years when friends would tout the value of eating properly, I would politely thank them and continue on my own destructive way. Never in a 'zillion' years, would I have dreamed that I would be writing this book. But here I am writing it! Please don't put it down. It could well save your life!

CHAPTER 6

THINGS THAT KILL

I have discovered that certain speeding items truly do kill. Take for example a speeding bullet that hits a person in their 'kill zone'. This includes the head and the upper torso of the human body. A bullet hitting someone in their kill zone, usually does just that, it kills them! One of the basic lessons when teaching firearm safety is to never point the gun at someone or something you do not wish to kill. Many indigenous peoples have learned to kill with darts or arrows dipped in some type of poison. If the arrow doesn't get you the poison will! The only real choice you have is to die quickly or to die over a longer period of time.

A SPEEDING TRAIN
As a young boy, I used to place pennies on the railroad track immediately in front of an oncoming train. Once the engine passed over the penny, it would fall to the ground flattened into a much different shape. Likewise, if you step in front of a speeding train, you probably will be killed.

Even though a train can flatten a penny, no train can stop on a dime! You also will be flattened in a rather dramatic fashion! That's certainly one way to make the headlines in the morning newspaper. You will have accomplished instant notoriety at a rather steep price.

A FAST AUTOMOBILE

If you are foolish enough to ride in a speeding automobile, you are at a substantial risk to be killed in a crash. Really, it makes no difference if you are driving the vehicle or simply a passenger. Either way, if you're dead, you're dead! Now I realize that all of us are someday going to be dead, but why rush the obvious? If you are a passenger in the speeding automobile you have several choices. You can ask the driver to slow down and drive more carefully. If this fails to convince him, you can ask the driver to stop and let you out. As a last resort, you can reach out and remove the key from the ignition, thereby bringing the car to a stopped and safe condition. Getting out and taking a walk certainly beats getting squished and ending up in the obituary column of next week's paper.

ARTERY ROADBLOCK

Plaque buildup in your arteries is equally as dangerous as a speeding bullet, a speeding automobile, or an oncoming train. Almost every modern city has underground storm drains installed to remove excess water during a storm. These are installed to prevent flooding. The wise leader of the city maintenance crew will make sure his crew takes time to clean the drains of leaves and debris during dry weather. Then when the rains come the drains work as intended. Plugged up drains cause flooding. We all know that flooded roads can be dangerous.

The circulatory system in our bodies works much the same way. Keep the arteries healthy and free from plaque buildup and the blood flows as intended. Not keeping them clean leads to much trouble. When a chunk of plaque breaks loose inside your artery, it can do great damage in a matter of seconds. It can break loose and form a road block, cutting off the supply of blood to your heart. If left untreated this will either greatly damage or destroy your heart muscle. This is called a myocardial infraction, also known as a heart attack. It has been documented that nearly half of both men and women die as a result of that first heart attack! Plaque can also form a roadblock stopping the blood from reaching your brain. This results in damage or death to the affected parts of your brain. We have a convenient term for this called 'having a stroke'. I've got news for everyone; if the brain dies, you die! Any way we look at it, blood clots are not fun! Both heart attacks and strokes can severely limit your quality of life if they do not kill you! Strokes can rob you of your memory as well as the ability to think logically. They can severely limit your ability to walk and even how and if you can carry on a conversation. I think the word we are looking for is 'Debilitating'. A stroke can completely ruin your chance to live a normal, happy life.

TAKING CONTROL

Thankfully, God has given every one of us freedom of choice. We were never created to function as robots. Throughout life we find speed bumps, speed traps, potholes and sometimes disasters! Speed bumps are placed in a road bed in order to slow down traffic. Speed traps are set up by law enforcement in order to prevent speeding drivers from causing harm to themselves or others. Speed disasters, on the other hand, are the results of one or more drivers ignoring their responsibility to keep themselves and others safe. As is the case with road conditions, so is the care and upkeep of the major blood vessels in our body. If we keep them clean and healthy, we have an excellent chance of living out our lives with little or no major issues with our blood circulation. When our blood is circulating properly, All the other organs of the body tend to also function properly. Our life and health are truly dependent on our healthy blood circulation.

CHAPTER 7

VEGGIES WITH VALOR

I'm sure glad that fruits and veggies along with nuts and seeds make up the largest part of my new style of eating. This, combined with regular exercise, is responsible for healing my heart and reversing my diabetes. This chapter is my attempt to correlate some of these 'happy heart' individual fruits, nuts and vegetables with desirable spiritual qualities. The Bible is very clear that our physical bodies and our Spiritual condition are closely related. Here are just a few examples of this from the book of Proverbs: "A glad heart makes a happy face; a broken heart crushes the spirit" (Proverbs 15:13). "A wise person is hungry for truth while the poor feeds on trash" (Proverbs 15:14). "A bowl of soup with someone you love is better than steak with someone you hate" (Proverbs 15:17). "A dry crust eaten in peace is better than a great feast with strife" (Proverbs 17:1). We could continue this study, but I'm sure you are starting to get the idea of this correlation. This chapter is my attempt to have some fun connecting spiritual values with some of the healthy fruits and vegetables I now enjoy with great 'regularity', (pun intended).

APPLES

Apple juice, applesauce, and especially apple pies are delicious inclusions to my heart healthy diet. Apples trees thrive from a periodic frost in order to get ready for the new crop of delicious apples. There are many types of apples around the world. While they are different shapes sizes and colors, they all have one thing in common. For an Apple tree to be productive the climate needs to have regular seasons which include at least one hard frost per year. Christians also need, and indeed thrive on periods of spiritual coldness. Spiritual coldness (or challenges) can be self-induced when we step back from our close relationship with God. Or at times it can be a period of testing from God. Every time we are tested we have the opportunity to grow 'new branches' which will in turn produce much more fruit. Owners of commercial orchards help this process along by pruning back the larger branches to encourage new growth, which in turn produces a greater crop of apples. In our spiritual life, we may be able to equate a larger branch with a bit of spiritual pride. God often needs to prune back our pride so that He can use us to produce useful spiritual fruit. Pride can be such an insidious force of evil. If we're not careful we can become proud of the fact that we have no pride! Listen to God's warning: "Pride goes before destruction and a puffed-up spirit before a fall" (Proverbs 16:18-19) kjv.

AVOCADOS

There are some vegetables, like avocados, which require a warm climate in which to thrive. Many Christians also need the warmth and security of a loving church family. This is good! There's nothing wrong with that! The avocado is a tree that is native to South Central Mexico. This is a warm, inviting climate. Technically the avocado is considered to be a fruit containing a single seed. Personally, it seems much more like a vegetable to me. Perhaps this is because it has such a yummy green texture to the fruit. It's hard for me to compare an avocado to a peach or a plum. The avocado is covered with a dark green skin that's all bumpy and full of wrinkles. In fact, from the outside it looks quite ugly. But, when you cut it open and scoop out the pit, you find a smooth, creamy, delicious flesh inside that is also very good for you. Yes, my friend, avocados are much like people. Many of us are not exceptionally beautiful on the outside, but like the avocado, this does not really matter! It's what's inside that counts! It's what's inside that truly determines the real you. When a stranger looks inside your 'skin' what do they find?

ARTICHOKE

This weird vegetable somehow reminds me of an armadillo. In my humble opinion, both the armadillo and the artichoke are just plain ugly! They are both covered with flat or semi-rounded little pieces of armor-like plating. At first glance, it seems like there is nothing edible about this thorny looking creation. I'm told that a small portion of flesh, hiding under the scales, is really quite delicious. My wife has tried, without much success, to turn me into a connoisseur of the lowly artichoke. It seems the only way to enjoy one is first you have to boil the heck out of it. Then, after it is softened up, you need to peel back each little plate of armor and scrape out the tiny bit of edible flesh from the underside. I'm told it's quite a delicacy. However, this vegetable lover would be quite content if God decided to 'rapture' all artichokes on the planet! Then, if He did this, we might be subject to a diet of artichokes when we get to heaven!

ASPARAGUS

Asparagus has many strange characteristics. If you plan on growing your own, the plant should be purchased in 'bare-root' form and planted early in the spring. Each individual plant normally consists of one single spear that grows up out of the earth once a year and lasts for a few short weeks. For the first two years, these spears should not be harvested. They are just too skinny and cutting them will rob the roots of needed nutrients. Usually by the third year the plant has matured sufficiently and the spears can be harvested. Each individual plant consists of one single spear that grows up once a year for a few short weeks That's all folks! Just one stalk! Once every year! Pretty much lying dormant for the rest of the season. You might think it's not worth it. However, there is a plus side. That one stalk tastes incredibly delicious! It is also very good for you! Another thought, every year the asparagus root sends forth a new stalk, bigger and better than the year before. It reminds me of each one of us growing in our Christian faith.

There are times when it takes an incredible amount of patience and effort for the Christian to build bridges of friendship with a non-Christian in order to be a witness. Let me assure you that every single person you meet is worth the time and effort needed to build a relationship. Often this is necessary before a non-believer will take you seriously. In God's eyes, every person is worth saving. Jesus came to earth and died to save those who were lost. The first time you lead a person to Christ you will experience incredible joy! Worth far more than waiting to taste a spear of asparagus! Every vegetable is different. The same can be said for every person! Did you know that all of Heaven rejoices when one single person gives their life to God through belief in Jesus Christ? (Luke 15:7).

BEANS
Test yourself, how many different kinds of beans can you name? There are green beans, yellow string beans, garbanzo beans (chickpeas), kidney beans (dark red, pink, white), black beans, navy beans, pinto beans, cannellini beans, lima beans, and soybeans just to name a few. To be honest, beans are some of the staples of my new diet. Beans are some of the most heart-healthy veggies ever created. There is no such thing as a bad bean! Sad to say, beans have suffered a terrible reputation among some people. It is true they can give you gas. Here comes the good news; they are high in protein, loaded with fiber, and have many other beneficial ingredients. Toss a can of garbanzo beans in the blender, add a few spices and perhaps some lemon juice and you have instant humus. This becomes a delicious spread on crackers or bread and even as a dip for raw veggies. Beans are truly some of my best friends. Speaking of friends, God has made many of my human friends equally diverse in size, shape, color and ethnic backgrounds. Jesus died for every person. He died for every man, woman or child, who will turn to him. His invitation is open to everyone of us!

I suspect that Jesus will not be recognized in heaven by many people who do not come from a Middle Eastern background. If you are looking for a blond haired, blue-eyed Jesus, you may be greatly disappointed. One thing is for certain, He will never disappoint you!

BEETS

Perhaps you never knew that beets are a wonderful source of nitric oxide! Nitric oxide (NO) has recently been discovered to have a powerful influence on our health and well-being. Nitric oxide is a gas which is formed when enzymes are broken down into an amino acid called L – Arginine which will aid in improving strength, enhancing recovery and even in muscle building. Beets are even referred to as the natural enhancement food to help athletes perform at an accelerated pace! Beets are good for you! Beets taste good! Beets help you to be your very best at any physical activity. Who wouldn't want to be a consumer of beets! Beets may be eaten as a yummy fresh vegetable. Beets can be used as a garnish to a salad. Beets can even be pickled and eaten as a relish. Nitric oxide derived from beets might even be compared to the Holy Spirit of God being fused into his people to empower them to do their very best for God. Beets have the ability to bleed their red color. Beet juice has been used to die cloth in many cultures. This helps to remind us of the blood Jesus shed to wash away our sins.

BROCCOLI

How many times has a child been told "Eat your broccoli, it's good for you!" It seems that broccoli is the king of all green vegetables! A stalk of broccoli even looks somewhat like a king including the large crown at the top. Broccoli is in the family of cruciferous vegetables along with cabbage and cauliflower. When I make Jesus my king, He makes me the instrument of his blessing with far more healing power than a stalk of broccoli!

BRUSSELS SPROUTS

All I can say about Brussels Sprouts is that they are baby cabbages. I have no idea why God made baby cabbages that don't taste as good as big cabbages! Perhaps it's because they are filled with nutrients, including folate, manganese, vitamin B6, dietary fiber, choline, copper, vitamin B1, potassium, phosphorus and omega-3 fatty acids. So much goodness in such tiny little heads! It may be that God uses these tiny heads to remind us not to allow our pride to give us a "swelled head".

CABBAGE

While cabbage has many beneficial qualities, it can also give you gas! This reminds me of some people. Perhaps this is where the term 'cabbage-head' comes from. It's also rich in vitamins A and C. Even when we are considered 'ordinary' in the eyes of others, every person has equal value in the eyes of God!

CARROTS

Carrots are known to parents as a food to make children see better. Children are often told to eat their carrots so they can see. There is some truth to this. Carrots contain a form of Vitamin A called Beta-Carotene which helps the Retina and other parts of the eye to function smoothly. In a similar fashion, reading God's word helps us to see more clearly his love and purpose for our lives.

CAULIFLOWER

One only needs to look at a head of cauliflower to be reminded that God has a wonderful sense of humor. It looks somewhat like a bleached-out brain. Sort of like it could belong to bones found out in the desert. Petrified grey-matter left behind by some thoughtless wanderer? I guess it's good for something!

CORN

Corn is one of the main staples of the civilized world. It ranks right up there with wheat and rice and beans. Corn can be dried and ground into flour (cornmeal). It can be roasted or boiled and eaten straight off the cob. It is the foundation for many packaged cereals such as cornflakes. It is also used as the basis for certain types of animal feed. Corn is primarily a crop native to the Western Hemisphere. Just like many happy people, corn tastes good and is good for you. It is pleasing to the eye and to the pallet. We need to practice becoming more like corn and less like cauliflower! Corn husks and corncobs have also been used for many needs. I believe that corn is a gift to us from the early Native Americans of North America. It's early origin possibly dating back 7,000 years to people who lived in present day Mexico. Thank you, friends!

CUCUMBERS

When is a cucumber not a cucumber? When it becomes a pickle! Just like some people, pickles can be either sweet or sour. Please make sure you do not become the sour type.

DANDELIONS
I may be one of the few people who has actually eaten dandelions! Trust me, they are not tasty! They are often tough to chew and almost always bitter. Eating dandelions is better than starving, but not that much better! However, they are free. You can dig them out of most anybody's front lawn. Items that are free are not always desirable. So be careful!

GRAPEFRUIT
Several 'cousins' to the grapefruit are very good for you. Lemons and Oranges are filled with Vitamin C. Grapefruit, when combined with certain medications, CAN BE DEADLY! Therefore, do your homework. Always understand the do's and don'ts of combining certain foods with grapefruit. We need to be aware that certain innocent acting persons can also be just as deadly. Scripture tells us to test the spirits to determine if they are from God. (1 John 4:1).

KALE
Kale is one of the most densely nutritious plants on the planet. High in vitamins, filled with minerals and omega 3. It helps protect against high blood pressure, depression, cancer, inflammation and heart disease. What a powerhouse of health from one vegetable!

LEEKS
Leeks remind me of giant sized green onions also known as scallions. As part of the onion family they are nutritious as well as delicious. Leaks are a pleasant addition to almost any recipe. Leaks have many of the good qualities found in

other members of the onion family including the antioxidant polyphenols.

LETTUCE

What would a salad be like without lettuce? Iceberg lettuce forms a head with many layers of goodness. But there are many other varieties such as green leaf lettuce, romaine lettuce, as well as red leaf lettuce, just to name a few. Lettuce is indeed, the foundation of most salads. Much the same as the leaves (pages) of the Bible are the foundation of the Christian faith.

MUSHROOMS

Mushrooms are a fungus. Some are delicious while others can be poisonous and even deadly. They can either taste heavenly or they can send you on an unscheduled heavenly adventure! They can give you joy or they can give you gout! Mushrooms are one of the few vegetables that prefer to grow and live in darkness. Sadly, some people also fit this description! Like so many other things in life, mushrooms need to be carefully tested and evaluated.

ONIONS

Why, O why, does an onion make you cry? They taste so good, yet often misunderstood. Only the brave can eat them raw. The more you remove the outer skin, the sweeter they become. Quite like some people. When we discover their inner sweetness, it brings moisture to our eyes. Sweet onions and sweet people are very much alike.

PEANUTS

When is a nut, not a nut? Most obviously, when it is a peanut. True nuts grow on trees. A peanut is in fact a legume also known as a 'ground nut' because it grows beneath the ground. One of the most popular names is 'goober'. Goober is derived from "nguba", the name for peanut in the Bantu language spoken in parts of Africa. Now you are an expert in the folklore of the peanut. Peanuts are a great source of protein as well as healthy oil. A "P B & J" sandwich could even be classified as a 'comfort food' for many children. And God knows that we all need a little bit of His comfort from time to time!

PEAS

The correlation of peas and protein is synonymous with hot and cold, or hard and soft. Peas are a great source of protein, and pea protein is a building block for many vegetarian diets. Peas have also been known to cause gout. Peas are like some people I have known. Some make you strong while filling you with lots of energy. But we need to be aware that too much of a good thing (or a person) can have unpleasant consequences! We may become too dependent on others for our strength. Personally, I like to look to God for my greatest source of energy and direction. He never causes harm or lets you down! You will never get a sore toe from walking with the Lord!

PEPPERS –

RED OR YELLOW, ORANGE OR GREEN - MOST ARE MELLOW, BUT SOME ARE OBSCENE. Filled with flavor and full of good stuff. Bell peppers can also be deliciously 'stuffed'. Some have reputations of being too hot to handle…much like certain types of humans. At one time, I was offered a taste of a Vallecito Pepper. This was by far the most painful bite into a vegetable that I ever experienced! My eyes watered and my nose ran! My mouth and throat reminded me of this for hours to come! This was indeed a most painful learning experience! People or peppers can both become labeled as 'HOTTIES'. Some can inflict great pain. So be careful!

POTATO

Russet or Redskin they all have delicious white insides and yummy, healthy skins. Filled with potassium and other important minerals. Potatoes can help lower your blood pressure. They are filled with phytochemicals and antioxidants. Recently, British scientists at the Institute for Food research, have discovered that potatoes contain another antihypertensive compound, kukoamines, which work like prescription ACE inhibitors and are so rare they have never been found in any other food! I find it interesting how many ways the potato can be prepared. Baked Potato is by far the most favored. Except perhaps for Hash Browns or French Fries. And let's not forget the lowly plain old boiled potato that is included in a huge variety of soups and stews and hash, and so many other combinations. The potato is perhaps one of the most versatile of all vegetables. It rivals pasta, beans and rice as a main staple food source in parts of the world. The potato reminds me of the average working-class wage earner. They may not be as glamorous as some vegetables, but try cooking for any amount of time without them! Average people are never considered as 'average' in the eyes of God!

We are the basic ingredient for everything God is accomplishing in this world!

PUMPKIN SEEDS

Pumpkin seeds and most seeds in general are filled with all sorts of goodies that are beneficial for our wellbeing. God made them that way for a purpose. Seeds have all the building blocks of their respective plants for their next generations! This reminds me of the poem "Trees". It states that "Poems are made by fools like me, but only God can make a tree." Do your research and find out those seeds that are healthy for you. Then practice eating them for pleasure and good health. Did you ever stop to think, that without seeds, there probably would not be a tomorrow! Only the reproductive power of God can cause a tiny seed to sprout become a living organism.

POMEGRANATE

Little tiny red berries clustered inside the outer skin of the fruit. Tiny in size but they pack a powerful punch against many diseases that would threaten us. They prevent the free radicals from attacking us. They fight cancerous cells by containing a uniquely powerful antioxidant called punicalagin. This is perhaps the most powerful antioxidant known to man.

PEACHES

Two of the more common types are known by the manner that the single seed, known as the peach pit, bonds with the fruit. These are called either 'cling' peaches or the 'free-stone' variety. This characteristic could be used to distinguish between two types of Christian believers. In this analogy, the pit becomes the person and the peach represents God. Do we cling to God in each situation or do we seek to be free and able to separate ourselves from Him whenever it seems convenient? I sincerely believe that God wants us to be clinging to him at all times!

RICE
Rice is the main food staple for a large percentage of the world's human population. It is easy to grow and it stores well for long periods of time. It cooks quickly in almost any container that can hold water and survive heat. Rice, in its natural state, is an excellent source of protein, carbohydrates and fiber. It is easily digested and combines well with most other foods. Wouldn't it be great if all people could become as easily and purposefully useful as the simple kernel of rice? The only requirement for a Christian to be useful is for us to be soaked, immersed in the power of God's Holy Spirit. At this point we are soft and pliable and willing to be used-up by God.

SPINACH
As a child, I remember the 'Popeye the Sailor' cartoons. I remember watching with amazement as this skinny sailor man would simply squeeze open and inhale a can of spinach, instantly becoming the most powerful guy around. Spinach is indeed filled with Iron and other beneficial vitamins and minerals. One of the problems is that the taste isn't the greatest! Mothers often combine it with something else more flavorful to trick the kids into 'eating their spinach'. When offering help to others, we need to be careful

not to become distasteful to them while offering our assistance. Never overwhelm someone with the power of God's presence.

SQUASH

Some people have asked how I keep from getting bored while just eating vegetables. One of the examples I tend to use pertains to the variety of squash available to us. The average person will tell you there are two types of squash. They will go on to name summer squash and winter squash as if these were self-inclusive varieties. Let me suggest that quite the opposite is true. In the summer squash variety, we have yellow squash, crooked-neck squash, and the most beloved zucchini in all of its different varieties. But did you know there are as many as 11 different types of winter squash? These begin with the little acorn squash and continue in size all the way to the huge Blue Hubbard squash. My daddy raised a Blue Hubbard squash that weighed 56 pounds and took the first prize blue-ribbon at the Connecticut State Fair one year. Now that's a squash to brag about! I suspect there are enough varieties of squash to satisfy most anyone's pallet!

SWEET POTATO

What is the difference between a sweet potato and a yam? Most people in the United States and other industrialized nations have never seen a true yam. Yams are native to Africa and parts of Asia. They do not grow in the United States. Yams are related to lilies, and can be as small as a regular potato or ridiculously jumbo in size. Some grow 5 feet long! The obvious question is, why do we have two types of sweet potatoes offered in many grocery stores in the United States? The obvious answer is that there are two main types of sweet potato. The 'firm sweet potato' has a golden skin and a pale-yellow flesh. While the 'soft sweet potato' as a copper colored skin and a deep orange colored flesh. Most grocery stores differentiate the 'soft sweet potato' by calling it a yam. Hopefully this information causes you to have a great deal of self-confident expertise among vegetarians! As a convention, you could really 'Yam' it up.

TOMATO

This chapter would never be complete without the tomatoes we love to eat. Tomāto or Tomăto, it's all the same to me. No matter how you say it, they make food taste so 'yummy'. Tomato ketchup is a staple for most American households. Some folks have been known to literally cover everything with ketchup until the only taste left is that of tomatoes. What would spaghetti or pizza be without tomato sauce? If you were to remove tomatoes, all salsa would be lost. They always make a salad taste it's very best. Without tomato sauce for pasta, the boot-shaped nation of Italy would surely starve to death! God has used tomatoes to make the world feel blessed!

VEGETABLE SOUP

Obviously, this is a combination of many different vegetables. I must confess that my homemade vegetable soup is by far my favorite meal. First and foremost, there is no right or wrong way to do it. No ingredients are more important than the other. Whatever I have, I use. I try to include as many different varieties as I have available. Raw and frozen

ones need to be cooked first. Liquid needs to be saved. I try
to include several cans of beans to every pot of soup, adding protein and fiber. When the whole big pot full has been
cooked, it then needs to be blended. I mean truly blended!
When vegetable soup has been run through the blender for
a sufficient amount of time, there is no possibility to ever
again differentiate one vegetable from the other. They are
all truly blended! My soup has literally become a sum of all
its parts. I believe this is God's plan for his church! I believe
this is God's plan for all humanity. I am absolutely certain
that God does not look upon us as people of different races,
nationalities, color or creed. God made us all, and he made
us all equal. He loves us all equally. God wants to bless his
people together while Satan wishes to drive us apart. Let's
determine not to let this happen!

WHOLE-WHEAT

I had a friend named Ned who was a member and for-
mer Chief of the Yavapai - Apache Reservation in Central
Arizona. He had a funny, weird sense of humor! Ned once
told me this story that he claimed was handed down from
his daddy: "There are four things that will kill you; white
salt, white sugar, white flour, and white men!" Whole-wheat
is simply wheat in its natural state. Before the grain has
been separated from its hull or its outer covering. The hull
is what gives it the distinct brown color along with many
nutrients and beneficial fibers. It seems rather foolish to remove the most beneficial part of the seed in order to call it
refined. Removing the hull has made the rice easy to cook,
but far less beneficial for our bodies. Then the food industry
tries to fool us by claiming this to be "fortified" with certain

added vitamins. They fail to mention the fact that the most beneficial outer hull or bran had been removed from the wheat kernel in the first place. Anything for a profit! I know a Jewish carpenter who once said, "The lusting after money is the root of all that is evil" (1 Timothy 6:10).

WALNUTS
Walnuts are a natural plant-based source of the beneficial oil we call omega-3. Walnuts are good for us and can be a delightful addition to many baked goods. Walnuts have one disadvantage. Since they contain oil, they do not store as well as other nuts. One trick to keep them from becoming rancid is to store them in the freezer. Christians need the fellowship of others so that our spirit can remain sweet and useful to God. Never let the enemy 'freeze' us out of a useful place in the army of God!

CHAPTER 8

STRESS IS NOT YOUR FRIEND

THOU SHALT NOT SWEAT IT

Worry not–Stress not. Worry and stress are closely related. Sort of like first cousins. There are two kinds of stress, the physical kind and the emotional type. It makes little difference whether you are suffering physical or emotional stress, the results are very similar. Stress is stress no matter in what form we find it. Medical gurus tell us that stress is a subtle, although a very significant killer of the human body! In the early years of my ministry I coined the phrase, "Thou shalt not sweat it". Somewhat, with tongue in cheek, I named this the 13th Commandment. Let's face it, worry, anxiety, fear are all gifts from the Devil. Each one of these is a gift which keeps on giving. In other words, once we become captivated by any one of these insidious gifts, Satan uses them to load us down with huge amounts of stress. God wants us to live a life of victory. Satan wants us to live a life of diminishing returns. Satan wants to burden us down with physical and emotional stress. Stress can lead to many negative conditions. It can rob us of sleep. This in turn can make us irritable and short tempered. Stress can really mess up a marriage. Stress can lead to a dysfunctional relationship with our Creator. Stress will definitely infringe upon my daily devotion time with God. If the Devil can keep me stressed out, I will also be tempted to "eat my frustrations". Or worse yet, to "drink my frustrations"! You don't have to be a rocket scientist to figure out where this is heading. The more I stress the more I eat. The more I eat the fatter I become. The more I gain in volume the more I lose in energy. In almost no time at all I am finding myself to be fighting the "Battle of the Bulge"! Satan wants me to use much of my energy in this fight. He also knows that my physical condition has a great deal to do with my Spiritual health. I've been told it's hard to love yourself when you hate your body. Stress also leads to discouragement. Stress can even cause physical illness which can lead to depression. We all know that depression can lead to thoughts of self-destruction. Stress can lower our sense of self-worth. The point of all this is that Satan is good at what he does. We dare not allow him to gain a foothold in our lives!

Let me present a two-part recipe to help remove stress in our lives:

LEARN TO PRAY EVERY DAY
Spend time with God. Get alone with God. Dare to get personal with God. Share with Him what's in your heart. Don't worry, He already knows everything about you! Tell him where you are struggling, and then ask Him for help in those areas. God is listening! God wants to help! All He's waiting for is for you to ask! There is no correct or wrong

way to pray. There is absolutely no need to include someone else in your prayer life. You do not need a religious leader to help you learn to pray. When Jesus died on the cross he opened the man-made barriers that separated each of us from God. In the Jewish Temple, there was a heavy curtain that divided the most holy place from the rest of the Temple. This was thought to separate the presence of God from the people of God. It was called the holy of holies. Jewish theology taught that only the high priest could go into the presence of God, and he could do this only once a year to plead for the sins of the people. This was one example of man-made rules and regulations. When Christ died on the cross, that curtain was torn from top to bottom! This signaled for all time that men and women could have free and complete access to God at any time and in any place. Scripture tells this plainly: "By this time, it was noon, and darkness fell across the whole land until 3 o'clock. The light from the sun was gone. And suddenly, the thick vail hanging in the Temple was torn apart. Then Jesus shouted, father I intrust my spirit into your hands! And with those words he breathed his last." (Luke 23:44-46)

LEARN TO PLAY EVERY DAY.
Sing and laugh and play and you'll drive the devil away! Playing makes us happy. Playing brings joy to our lives in all sorts of ways. It's hard to feel depressed when we're having fun! When we learn to play, we defeat Satan's plan to add stress to our lives. When we add aerobic exercise to our play, we defeat Satan yet another way. We give our body a chance to heal and get strong again. We discover how good it is to have fun. We overcome many of the

aches and pains brought about or intensified by our inaction. As one law of science says, "A body in motion tends to stay in motion unless acted upon by an opposite force". The opposite force, in this case, would be inaction. This would lead to another opposite force called depression. Depression is an insidious force of the devil! Depression can take an active, positive, person and turn them into a stagnant non-achiever almost overnight. Don't let depression sneak up on you!

Stress can hurt your body and your mind almost as much as a heart attack or stroke. Very little is written about stress related injuries or illnesses. Perhaps this is because stress conditions do not warrant the spending of huge amounts for research and development. Most doctors will tell you "Take two aspirin and call me in the morning". We all know that aspirin are cheap. They work rather well at a surprisingly low cost. We do not need a doctor to prescribe them. We do not need to worry about the government regulating them. While an aspirin may help to relieve the immediate symptoms, they only last a few hours. Figure out how you like to play. Find something you truly enjoy. Find one or more friends to play with you. At the very least, find a dog that likes to walk on his or her leash. They make wonderful companions. Dogs also know how to keep a secret. In fact, I've never known a dog to betray our confidence. They will love you when no one else does. Set up specific times on a regular basis for you and your friends to play. Please do not substitute electronic games for physical play! If you do, you will wear out your thumbs and still remain depressed!

DAMAGING EFFECTS OF STRESS
While surfing the Internet, I found research relating to why stress is the most dangerous toxin in our life. I never thought of stress as a toxin before, but this makes sense. Stress is well known but little understood. Stress is difficult to measure. If it can't be identified with a specific cause and effect it is often dismissed as not being 'real'. The article goes on to state specific ways stress is possibly the most dangerous toxin your body faces every day.

Stress confuses how our genes express themselves.
The chemicals your body produces when you are under stress turns on or off the genes that determine everything from how much fat you store, to how well your system works, to how fast you age, to whether or not you will develop cancer. Stress confuses these genes and therefore determines bizarre reactions in our bodies.

Early life experiences can influence your trigger point for stress.
Many times, a person tenaciously remembers good and bad experiences from their early childhood. Research shows that very early childhood events set your corticotropin releasing hormone. Consequently, any high or low level of this stress relieving hormone is capable of adjusting your adrenals and therefore your stress levels.

Stress often causes brain damage.
High level of stress hormones damage critical parts of the brain, such as the hippocampus, the area responsible for

memory. One reason people experience adrenal burnout after long-term chronic stress, is because the brain, in order to save itself, turns off the adrenals. We don't really know how much long-term damage this can cause.

Stress slows the immune system and increases inflammation.
Stress can be responsible for slowing wound healing, diminishing the protective effects of vaccines, and increasing your susceptibility to **infections**. Stress is the cause of many immune system failures. Stress is even they thought aggravated the recurrence of latent symptoms such as bone infections.

Chronic stress damages your mitochondria.
These energy factories produce a current through which all cells and organs in your body work. The good news is this damage is reversible over time, as stress goes away.

Stress reduces your ability to metabolize and detoxify.
Studies have shown that the activity of hundreds of genes responsible for enzymes that break down fats and detoxify prescription drugs, are negatively impacted by stress. Stress can also increase your toxin burden by increasing your desire for high-fat, high-sugar foods. Hence, we have the saying, "eating away one's frustrations".

Your cardiovascular system responds to stress.
Stress increases your cardiac output. This can be helpful if you have to run away from a certain danger for a short period of time. But chronic or long-term stress has been shown to increase the thickness of the artery walls, leading

to high blood pressure and heart disease. Stress can adversely mess with your heart and artery functions. This certainly got my attention! Eating properly and reducing stress may be equally important to my quality and longevity of life! I never equated these two factors before! I'll bet you never did, either!

<u>Stress adversely impacts your sexual abilities.</u>
Chronic stress increases the production of cortisol, leading to a condition called cortisol steal, where fewer sex hormones are produced. This may even increase the stress level. Which in turn exacerbates your problems! It seems that stress and impotency are closely related. They certainly are not friends.

<u>Stress is harmful for your bones and muscles</u>.
There is evidence to suggest that higher stress levels are associated with lower bone mineral density. Many studies have shown that people under chronic stress experience more physical pain. Excess stress in your life, may indeed, give you a pain in the 'lower back'! Is it possible that stress can also make your bones more brittle?

<u>Stress causes you indigestion</u>
There is more and more research showing stress impacts the function of your stomach and intestines. Stress slows normal transit of food, leading to constipation and other complications. It increases the overgrowth of bad bacteria. And it loosens the barriers between the cells that line the intestines., that can lead to inflammation, food sensitivities and even autoimmune disease.

Hopefully we now can all agree that stress is not our friend! I suggest that if stress is not our friend it must be our enemy. Stress is not merely neutral. Too much stress can really mess you up! Stress can adversely affect you physically, emotionally, and spiritually.

VALUE OF REDUCING STRESS

When controlled by stress, your life becomes a mess. It may be considered an oversimplification to state that by removing stress we stand an excellent chance of improving the quality of our lives. Easy to say, difficult to accomplish! The following chapter will examine some of the means available to us to help reduce stress and therefore improve our lives.

CHAPTER 9

STRESS - BUSTERS

SET YOUR SIGHTS

Goals are good ways to measure success and progress. However, we must be careful not to let goals define who we are or what we can achieve. Goals must be our goals not someone else's. You are the one and only person who is allowed to set goals for your life! The only one allowed to set goals for you to accomplish, is you! Never allow yourself to get suckered in to someone else's ideas of who you are or who you should become. You set the rules! You set and change the goals as you see fit! Always remember this!

It's always important and helpful to understand that progress comes in small bunches. It never comes all at once. A child needs to learn to take baby steps before they can become a marathon runner.

Recently I was sitting in the waiting room of my friendly physician, waiting for my number to be called, when I noticed a little toddler who had escaped the clutches of his mother. This little guy was running around and around a low table covered with magazines. He would make three or four laps around the table, then he would stop, drop to his knees, and began to crawl. Then he would abruptly push himself back up onto his wobbly legs and begin to run again! The lesson he taught me was this: even though we want to run ahead, there are times when we need to stop and crawl a little while. Once we're rested, then it's okay to get up and run again.

If you are trying to build up your body strength and your goal is to accomplish a certain number of push-ups or chin-ups, who would in their right mind will tell you to go from 0 to 60 in just one month! Anyone knows that this takes time! If you're lucky, you start out with one or two. Then you gradually increase to three or four or five. Before long you'll be up to seven or eight or nine! It may take you six months before you can do 60. You may never get to 60! 60 may be a totally unreasonable goal for you considering your physical capability. If I were your physical trainer, I would strongly suggest evaluating your capabilities, your age, your weakness and your strength. Then and only then could you set reasonable goals for yourself. Lofty goals are just that, they are lofty goals. What good are goals if they may sound good but only lead to defeat, only lead to discouragement, which leads to depression. Trust me, you not want to go there! Depression is a very bad place to be! Make your goals reasonable. Make your goals achievable. Only then can you make yourself accountable to achieve your goals!

LEARN TO PUSH YOUR PLATE AWAY

How many times does a well-meaning mother tell her child to finish her dinner, or to clean her plate. Little do they know that over-eating causes all sorts of problems. Many parents use guilt to force their children to over eat. Such guilty statements as, "Think of all the starving children in China"! This is absolute foolishness! Children and adults should never be forced to overeat! This is just wrong! Our bodies are built in such a way as to signal the brain when we have filled the belly! In fact, studies have been made that indicate the size of the plate determines the size of the meal! People who eat from a smaller plate usually feel more satisfied with a smaller meal than those who eat from a large plate piled high with food. Small is good! Less is often more! An amazing fact is that a person who eats less eventually weighs less! No need to count calories! Much better to plan a 'push-away' of your plate! This can also improve your development of the triceps muscles in your upper arm!

WALK A MILE EVERY DAY
Walking is one of the most painless ways for almost anyone to get some good exercise. An older friend of mine, who certainly could be considered a senior citizen, carries a device known as a pedometer. This measures how many steps she takes each day. Her claim is that she walks at least 3 miles a day in the normal course of events. This may sound extraordinary to most of us. However, I may have failed to mention that she and her husband have adopted and are the caretakers for eleven handicapped children! If you live or work in a city, why not use the stairs instead of an elevator? Do you shop in a multilevel mall? Forget the escalator! When our oldest children were growing up we lived in a small town in the Sierra Foothills. Those poor deprived kids were utterly amazed when we went to 'the city' where they first discovered "moving stairs"!

GET UP
It is a given fact that couch potatoes do very little exercise. I've never known a couch potato to take a walk. The only exercise I know of for a couch potato is to roll over or possibly to

sit up! Some couch potatoes won't even wait upon themselves for their basic needs! They may train their dogs to get their slippers. They may train their wife to get their drinks. Some couch potatoes even become emotionally attached to their favorite couch! It seems they never want to leave it alone! What a sad way to live! The first step to rehabilitating a couch potato is to help them learn how to stand up and get focused. Life does look better from a standing position!

GET GOING

Once a couch potato separates themselves from their couch, the battle is only half-won. The next step is really huge! They need to take their first step! It's almost like teaching a newborn baby how to walk! Only this baby may weigh 200 pounds or more! If you make the mistake of letting the couch potatoes stand for too long, they may turn around and sit down once again! If you are fortunate enough to get them up, you need to get them going! For this you need a plan.

SHAKE A LEG

A wonderful plan is to convince any couch potato to take a walk. It doesn't need to be very long walk. I might suggest that it needs to be a walk outside of the house. Away from the couch. Possibly a walk with a specific destination may prove helpful. Remember, couch potatoes have an emotional attachment to their couch! We need to break that attachment at all costs. Once the couch potato begins to move there are all sorts of possibilities!

Walking, running, jogging and sprinting are all excellent ways to shake a leg and burn off calories. These are also excellent ways to improve muscle tone and lung capacity. This type of exercise also does wonders to improve our circulation, blood pressure and heart condition! The more ambitious persons might consider a short game of basketball or some other activity with anyone who is willing to help. Even a game of table tennis is better than lying on the couch! If at all possible, find a way to ride a bicycle. If you don't own one, perhaps you have a friend who will loan you a used one, taking up space in their garage. Find a used bike for sale. Find a bike riding partner or two to make it that much more fun!

To me, 'shake a leg' has a double meaning. First and foremost, I only have one leg! I proudly wear a prosthesis on my left leg. Yes, I do take it off at night! In my house at night, if someone hollers fire, I will have to jump out of bed and jump or hop in a 'one-legged' sprint to the nearest exit! Or, if I have enough time, I can put on my prosthetic leg and actually run for my life! Physical exercise can be a powerful tool to our health and well-being. Those of you with two legs have no excuse whatsoever!

ROW, ROW, YOUR BOAT

I love old songs. I love to sing old songs. One that comes to mind goes like this, "Row, row, row your boat gently down the stream. Merrily, merrily, merrily, merrily, life is but a dream." What happens if we're not rowing downstream? What happens if life has dealt us a really bad hand? What happens if all our rowing is upstream? Always rowing against the current! Never seeming to get ahead! What do we do then? First of all, we do not row in the center of the river, that's where the most resistance comes from! We try to row along the riverbank where the water is gentler. At times, we may reach out and grab a branch along the riverbank to stabilize our boat and rest from our rowing. This is totally okay! This makes lots of sense!

I have an old-fashioned rowing machine. I call this the "cardiac express". It's on this 'old girl', as I call her, that I channel most of my physical exercise. Since I find it difficult to walk any great distance, this machine has been my constant physical companion and my daily challenge. It gives me the opportunity to build my arm muscles, strengthen my back and give my legs a good workout all at the same time. It helps to build my stamina and to increase my heart health as well as my circulation. 10 months ago, I would struggle to accomplish 20 'rows' at one time. This was accompanied by heavy breathing. As my health improved so did my stamina. Today I can pull 150 'rows' without breaking a sweat or breathing hard. Physical exercise really does work. I will go so far as to claim that you cannot obtain good health without regular exercise. Try it, and make sure to figure out some way to make it fun! If it is not fun, it will soon become a drudgery. Who wants to work-out on something that you dread? Think outside the box. If you are financially able, why not join a local gym. Maybe invite a friend to join you. Lighten up and make it fun!

DISCIPLINE

One of the important lessons I learned as a candidate at Naval Officer Candidate School was a strong sense of discipline. We had to develop self-discipline at the highest degree of discipline required by the Navy, if we were to succeed and accomplish our goal. It is important to understand that we developed the discipline to accomplish the goal! The goal was the most important thing. The goal was to become naval officers. The goal was to accomplish this no matter what the cost! Those officer candidates who did not succeed were the men who would not pay the price to develop that self-discipline.

This book is about developing your healthy body, for your benefit, for the rest of your life. To accomplish this, you must develop your self-discipline! Self-discipline does not come easily! Self-discipline is never accomplished without some failure and some setbacks. The difference between the winners and the 'also-rans' is measured in the degree of self-discipline. The question is, how badly do I want to succeed? Self-discipline is similar in many ways to training for a race. The first question I would ask concerns the distance of the race. Is it a 100- yard-dash? Is it a 400-yard race with hurdles? Is it perhaps a 2-mile cross-country race? I believe the 'get healthy'- 'stay healthy' race is one that becomes a habit for the rest of your life! It has a beginning but not an end. A young pastor friend of mine is training for his first marathon. At this point in time he is at the ten-mile point of his training. He has his eyes fixed on the goal. He plans to run a marathon! Using this analogy, what is your goal for living out the rest of your life? Are you training for a short period of time? Let me emphasize this is your race of a lifetime! If you wish to be successful, once you start you will never be able to quit! It will be a new way of life, for the rest of your life! Studies show that for most folks, the first twelve weeks are the hardest. If you will stick with it for twelve weeks, your chances for continued success improve tremendously! Make a commitment to yourself to succeed in this!

HOW AM I DOING?

Most results happen in very small increments; therefore, it would be impossible to measure them if we did not have some reliable method to do just this. Many children as they are growing taller ask some adult to measure how

tall they are getting. Often a mark is made with a cor-
responding date on a wall or some other surface. Later
another mark is made on that same surface to record the
child's growth during the year. No responsible adult will
attempt to record the child's growth every week. Growth
just happens much too slowly. The same is true with
our physical health. Thankfully we do have measures
to record our progress. Your doctor can order blood
tests to determine such things as cholesterol levels and
blood sugar measurements which could indicate diabetes. They will also test you for blood pressure, pulse rate
and oxygen levels among many others. This is important
information for them to know. It is also extremely important that you know and understand the meaning of
these tests. These are measurable results for your benefit
as you watch your body improve and become healthier.
You might wish to keep some sort of a personal 'progress
journal' to measure your success. This can act as your
personal measure of improving excellence toward your
final goal of a healthy, satisfying life.

SPIRITUAL EXERCISES

QUIET TIME

Scripture says, "God is our refuge and strength, always
ready to help in times of trouble" (Psalm 46:1). "Be still
and know that I am God! I will be honored by every
nation. I will be honored throughout the world. The
Lord of heaven's armies is here among us; the God of

Israel is our fortress" (Psalm 46:10-11). "If God is for us, who can be against us?" (Romans 8:31).

These and many other verses, give us the assurance that we can totally rely upon the love of God in every situation. Therefore, instead of worrying or being frustrated or fearful, it is extremely helpful for us to start each day alone in the presence of God. Jesus offers us His Peace even in the midst of the storms of life.

> "Peace I leave with you. My peace I give unto you. Not as the world gives, give I unto you. Let not your heart be troubled, neither let it be afraid." (John 14:27) kjv.

> 'Quiet time' is exactly that. It is choosing to physically remove myself from the clamor of everyday life in order to get alone with God. In order to have the opportunity to allow God to speak to my heart. A quiet time and place where I can listen to the voice of God. In the Scriptures, we read that Jesus himself felt the need for just such an opportunity. "While it was still dark, Jesus got up, and went off to a solitary place, and there prayed" (Mark 1:35).

DAILY DEVOTIONS

It is equally important to spend quality time each day reading and studying the word of God. A Daily Devotion is an excellent way to get in the habit of studying God's word. It is also a special time to bring your needs and concerns before

God in prayer. Scripture promises that God listens to each of our prayers. He truly cares about you and me. God wants us to learn to trust him. He wants to spend quality time with each of his children. God is our loving spiritual father! It stands to reason that as such, God wishes for us to get to know Him better. Spending time with God in praise and worship is a perfect way to learn the heart of God our heavenly Father. It can be as short or as long as you desire. The most important idea is to develop the habit of daily Scripture reading, prayer and worshiping God.

KEEPING A JOURNAL

Keeping a journal is an excellent way to document the faithfulness of God. It can become a historical record of when God answers prayer. It can become a record to encourage others. A spiritual journal is much like a personal diary between you and God. Your journal can become like a drink of fresh water when you feel spiritually dry. Writing in your journal helps you to gain insight into what God is teaching you each day. It can become a record of God's blessings to help when those tiny thoughts of doubt creep in. Try it, you'll like it! Make your journal writing become a good habit. Like a record of your sweet times with God!

CHAPTER 10

REBUILD YOUR BODY

<u>YOUR LEAN MACHINE</u>

Why is it that we don't see many heavy people at the gym? You and I both know that heavy people are extremely sensitive about their looks and their weight. Whoever coined the term 'obese' certainly knew how to hurt a person! How much more damage can be done by using the term "morbidly obese"? Let's face it, if you fall into this category you are certainly not alone, but you may feel quite alone. Some 35% of the United States population was considered morbidly obese in the year 2015. Obesity seems to be a national disease that is constantly on the increase. Moreover, obesity seems to follow certain geographical patterns. According to the United States National Center for Health Statistics, <u>morbid obesity</u> is most highly concentrated in Louisiana, Alabama and West Virginia. The NCHS data shows that <u>obesity</u> is most highly concentrated east of the Mississippi River with the exceptions of Maine, Ohio, Virginia, and Florida. The same data indicates that Oregon is the only state west of the Mississippi with a high concentration of morbidity. All of the other populations in states west of the Mississippi are shown to be either slightly obese or within the realms of normality. There is a substantial increase in medical costs for citizens carrying extra pounds around their midsection's and the posterior portions of their anatomy! It seems that the estimate is for obese patients to cost $1,429 more per person, per year, on average, than the less portly members of society. This study shows that 36.5% of adults in the United States qualify as being obese. That's over one in three, folks!

Obesity related medical conditions include heart disease, stroke, type II diabetes and certain types of cancer. These are some of the leading causes of <u>preventable</u> death! Just these figures alone should motivate each one of us to honestly evaluate our stature by looking in the mirror, and stepping on the scales. Using a tape measure around the middle will help to confirm the results! This condition is one that can be controlled very simply if the obese person is willing to take control of their lifestyle! By this I do not mean going on a diet, purchasing expensive nutritional additives, or going on some crash course that promises to help us lose weight. One simple fact is that most obese people have one thing in common. They do not exercise! They do not walk. They do not run. They do not jog. Most of them do not own a bicycle. You won't find many of them on the ski slope. Nor will you find them on the basketball court. But where you will find them is on the couch or in their favorite chair. Hence the term "Couch Potatoes"! The most exercise many of these folks get is "Thumbing" on some electronic devise! Or changing TV channels with their remote. It's hard to believe that we have become so lazy that we consider it a chore to get up and walk across a room in order to physically change the channel we are watching!

Changing the way we eat, must, I repeat, <u>must</u> be coupled with an integrated exercise program. The way we eat and the way we move will combine to shape how we are "shaped"

There is a definite connectivity between the way we look and the way we feel! We cannot feel good about ourselves when we are ashamed of how we look. Unlike the hippopotamus or walrus, God did not create humans to be obese! We seem to have accomplished this all by ourselves! Starting your exercise program is easy! It only takes desire and determination.

Here is my honest opinion based upon personal experience and observation. Any obese person who **commits** <u>to a</u> **vegetarian lifestyle**<u> combined with moderate exercise</u> will continue to lose fat and gain lean muscle until they are no longer considered obese. At this point in time you will love your body and have the opportunity to love yourself more completely! If you choose to **commit** <u>to a</u> **vegan lifestyle** <u>with moderate exercise</u>, the change will happen that much quicker. Either way, the change will take place! How badly do you want it?

<u>PROTEINS ARE BUILDING BLOCKS</u>

Protein is the absolute essential ingredient needed for building and maintaining muscle strength. In the industrialized nations of the world we have been 'fed' the misconception that a protein sufficient diet <u>must</u> consist of red meat, eggs, and dairy products. Because of this, when considering protein in the diet, most people immediately think of meat, poultry and fish, along with eggs and dairy products. While it is true that these are all high in protein, we need to look at the possibility of ulterior motives. It appears that some of the persons who are responsible for recommending certain foods to the general public are also beneficiaries of the profits made by companies producing those same meat, poultry and dairy products that are being recommended. There appears to be a significant conflict of interest. If this indeed is true, how much credibility should the average person place on these "balanced nutritional pyramids" being promulgated in so many nutrition publications? It could be likened to asking the dairy farmer to evaluate the benefits of drinking milk for adults over the age of forty! Or the poultry industry having chicken farmers investigate the values of eating chicken three times a week. Just a thought!!

Protein is a component of every single cell your body. Some of the other foods that are high in protein include all types of beans, soy, whole grains as well as nuts and seeds. It is important to understand that a well-balanced vegetarian diet will supply all the protein needed for the average person. Now that is indeed enlightening!

BEANS, BEANS THE MUSICAL FRUIT

For those of us who have made the switch, and for those of you who are contemplating such a move, be confident that you can get an adequate amount of protein from fruits, nuts and vegetables, without the addition of meat, poultry, eggs and dairy products. This may come as a shock to many of you. When it comes to protein, beans are a man's best friend. The good news is, there are at least 17 varieties of beans that I am aware of. Even better news is that each of these varieties are extremely high in protein, fiber, and other wonderful nutrients. Plus, of course, we have the wonderful coffee beans, which truly are man's best friend! Drink more coffee and live longer and live better!

Unless you are extremely lazy, there is no such thing as a bland, tasteless, vegetarian diet! Some of the most wonderful cooks and chefs I have discovered work their culinary magic without the use of meat or foul or eggs or dairy products. These are the true culinary geniuses of our day! Their food is delightful while providing all the nutrients a body could want without all the damaging effects of processed foods, sugar and meat products.

STAMINA
Stamina, also referred to as endurance, has both a physical and a mental element involved. To increase one's stamina requires both training and mental focus. The benefits of physical stamina include better fitness levels along with a lower risk of heart problems as we increase our cardiovascular endurance. Athletes with strong stamina are able to compete for longer distances and for longer periods of time. Stamina allows your body to function at high levels despite the risk of pain, fatigue and stress. Perhaps because it's easier to maintain focus we tend to make fewer mistakes whether training for tough competition or simply a challenging workout. This also translates to our brainpower! You will perform better when your brain has this increase in blood flow. Contrary to some popular opinions, the brain is intricately attached to the body and is dependent upon the cardiovascular health of the heart and blood vessels.

One of the reasons we start to get absent-minded as we age is because many older people develop a hardening of the arteries. This in turn inhibits blood flow to the brain. The reduced blood flow to the brain results in slower brain functions including memory loss. This condition can be exacerbated when we suffer mini-strokes. Just one more reason to keep our blood vessels healthy.

PAIN REDUCTION

Almost everyone reaching the age of 50 is beginning to experience certain aches and pains in the muscles and joints. Arthritis has become your secret companion. Arthritis stays closer than your very best friend! It greets you in the morning when you first wake up! It hangs around most of the day and is especially personal when evening arrives. Arthritis is your one companion who will never leave you while you are on this earth! With this in mind, we do not have to let arthritis be our master! I have found that simple stretching and twisting exercises can do much to lessen the impact of my old acqaintance, Arthritis. Once again, I refer you to my rowing machine. It has the ability to stretch out the spaces between my vertebrae. This gives much needed relief to the 'squished' or compressed condition of the discs separating each member of my backbone! Relief is just a stretch or two away. Another ideal solution is to stand, and stretch, and touch your toes! This may even produce popping effects as your back seeks to realign itself. Do your back a favor and learn how to stretch!

STRETCH AND TWIST AND STRETCH
SOME MORE
DO IT LYING ON THE FLOOR
THEN JUMP UP AND STRETCH SOME MORE

CHAPTER 11

BUILDING SELF ESTEEM

Almost every bathroom I have ever entered features at least one mirror. Why is a mirror so important? We all wish to look our very best, especially when we are out in the public. It has been reported that the average woman spends over $200,000 on make-up and cosmetics during her lifetime. That's about as much as it would cost to buy the average house. Other studies claim the amount is closer to $300,000 over a woman's lifetime. One study claims that this averages out to approximately eight dollars a day just to make your face look good. It's no wonder that famous personalities spend huge amounts of money on such things as 'facelifts' and 'tummy tucks'. Most people agree, "if you want to feel good you need to look good"!

LOOK GOOD AND FEEL GOOD
It is much easier to feel good about yourself when the mirror tells you that you look pretty darn good! After all, mirrors never lie! Except when they are in a mirror fun-house

at the local carnival! When our body feels healthy, this translates, to an amazing degree, to how we look! We tend to stand up straight and to walk with a purpose. It's hard to slouch when you feel good about yourself! A 'feel-good' body often translates into a smile on the face. A smile on your face may often become contagious. Offer a smile and many times people smile back. A smile can even turn into a laugh or chuckle. "There's an old saying, "Laugh and the world laughs with you, cry and you cry alone". When you smile your face-muscles will thank you. They won't have to work as hard.

CHAPTER 12

WHAT IS MY BODY TELLING ME ?

There is absolutely no substitute for your gut feeling about any situation! Some folks call this intuition. Another term might be natural instinct. The truth is that our body is constantly and consistently sending us messages about its overall health and welfare. Our body also gives us specific messages that demand our immediate attention. Such as a toothache! Or a painful injury.

These are the type of message that we normally recognize and act upon immediately. But what about the many other messages that our body is sending us?

DANGER SIGNALS
God has designed our bodies to respond in certain ways when something is seriously wrong. One telltale message is how quickly we become short of breath during normal activities. Another message may be a loss of appetite. Or

a significant reduction in our energy level. We universally recognize the message associated with a deep cough or a rising body temperature. We also recognize the signs of a sudden pain in the chest accompanied by shortness of breath! This demands immediate attention with the probable rush to the nearest hospital. A potential heart attacks is something we take seriously. What about the message of aching joints? How much attention do we pay to arthritis? Our body may be calling attention to sudden weight loss. Or possible memory dysfunction which may be associated with mini-strokes. How important is it for you to listen to what your body is trying to tell you? It's early warning system may help you take appropriate action for a situation before it becomes serious. Lesson number one should be, that we listen to our bodies and understand what they are trying to tell us! When your body gives you a call, never put it on 'hold'! Answer that call and pay strict attention. It may save your life!

Guess what? Actions really do speak louder than words! When my body gives me a message, I need to act! If you receive a call that your house is on fire, you don't just thank the caller and go about your normal affairs. Anyone with half a brain will take immediate action! Get everyone to safety! Assess the immediate situation! Decide on a plan of action! Above all, follow through and take the appropriate action! All the careful planning in the world is useless unless it is followed by action! Women are so much smarter in this area. If the truth be told, women are much smarter than men in almost every area! The secret to why women generally live longer than men is that they are willing to take action when action is called for! Most women are not too proud to go to the doctor when they note that something is wrong. On the other hand, many men wait far too long to even admit something may be wrong. Since I am a man, I can get away with saying that a majority of men are truly short sighted in this area!

SCHEDULED MAINTENANCE

Proper maintenance of any machine dictates that we have a regular scheduled maintenance on all the moving parts. Who would buy a new car and fail to change the oil and perform regular service of that new car? Nobody in their right mind would be so foolish! Our bodies are just like any other machine. They are living, moving machines that also need to be maintained. What's good for any other machine should also be good for the living machine in which we live. A chiropractic friend of mine has a sign in his office which reads: "If you don't take care of your body, where on earth will you live?" Think about it! We might also reflect on the fact that for a Christian, our body is the temple, the dwelling place, of God's Holy Spirit! "Don't you know that your body is the temple of the Holy Spirit..." (1 Corinthians 6:19). This fact alone should make us want to maintain our body in tip top shape.

CHAPTER 13

WHAT ARE THE LAB TESTS
TELLING ME ?

Hopefully, you are not the type of person who resists going to a doctor or spending the money to have lab tests. Hopefully you are not the type of person who simply 'knows' that you are feeling fine. The type of person who refuses to 'make doctors rich'! The type of person who does not really believe in preventive medicine. The person who boasts he has never been sick a day in his life. This is also the type of person who does not have a clue if there is anything wrong with his health. I hope you will thank God that you are not this type of person! We need our doctor much more than he needs us!

Every adult should make it a habit to have a physical checkup at least once a year. This is true especially when you know there is nothing wrong with you. Most doctors will order certain tests to be performed before your annual visit. One such test is a full panel blood test. This will test for proper function of your major organs as well as levels of important areas of blood chemistry. A blood panel may also point out any areas of concern such as diabetes or abnormal functioning of the liver and kidneys. A urinalysis is also a normal part of this evaluation. These tests were not available in your grand-parents lives, but they are available to you today. It's interesting to note that the average lifespan of earlier generations was about half of what it is today! Yes, my friend, lab tests have a great deal to do with this! If you are afraid of the needle, you might ask a friend to hold your hand to give you courage to face the phlebotomist! If you don't like the site of your own blood, don't look! Many lives have been saved because of the early warning provided by a blood test.

I have been rushed to a hospital seven times for suspected heart attacks. Each time a blood test has been used to verify that a heart attack was indeed happening. During a heart attack part of your heart is dying. As if crying for help, it emits a certain protein enzyme into the blood. A simple blood test can instantly identify that your heart is dying and screaming for help. The wise man or woman does not wait for this to happen. The wise person listens to their body on a regular basis. The wise person seeks to prevent heart attacks and other serious illness by the way we treat our body. For the first 77 years of my life, I was not a wise person. In the last three years this has changed radically. I now qualify as a wise person in this area. Are you a wise person?

CHAPTER 14

WHAT ARE THE ENDURANCE TESTS TELLING ME ?

DOCTOR ORDERED STRESS TESTS

One of the standard tests to measure the strength and overall health of our heart is called the cardiology stress test. Cardiac stress test measures blood flow to your heart at rest and while your heart is working harder as a result of exertion while running on a treadmill. This physical act of running can also be accomplished with medication for those who cannot perform on the treadmill. The test provides images that can show areas of low blood flow through the heart and damaged heart muscle. The test usually involves taking two sets of images of your heart. One while you are at rest and another after your heart is stressed, either by exercise or medication.

You may be given a nuclear stress test. This involves injecting a radioactive dye into your bloodstream. This may be ordered if your doctor suspects you have coronary artery disease or if a routine stress test did not pinpoint the cause of symptoms such as chest pain or shortness of breath. A nuclear stress test may also be useful to guide your treatment if you've been diagnosed with a heart condition. If you have symptoms that might indicate coronary artery disease, such as shortness of breath or chest pains, nuclear stress test can help determine if you have coronary artery disease. It may help your doctor see the size and shape of your heart. Images from a nuclear stress test can show your doctors if your heart is enlarged, and can measure its pumping function [ejection fraction].

A nuclear stress test may also be a useful guide in the treatment of heart disorders. If you been diagnosed with coronary artery disease, arrhythmia, heart valve dysfunction, or another heart condition, nuclear stress test can help your doctor find out how well your treatment is working. It may also be used to help establish the right type of exercise for you by determining how much exercise your heart can safely handle.

SELF-TESTING
Self-testing should only be done in addition to endurance tests administered by your doctor. Your body will give you feedback if you are able to listen and properly interpret what you are being told. How well is your body tolerating a particular type of exercise? Is your body comfortable with improving the quality of exercise or the length of time for any one exercise? Are your muscles rebelling or rebuilding? Are your lungs comfortable with your type of exercise? Are all your joints compatible with what you're asking them to

accomplish? It is super important that we listen to our body! Life is not good when we allow our body to wear out.

Several months ago, my 24-year-old son decided that he wished to become a physical trainer. He determined that he needed to make several adjustments to his physical body in order to become a believable example to any potential clientele. He went on a self-imposed diet combined with a personalized physical regimen. Now, several months later, he is fit and trim and feeling really good about himself! He did the research, made the commitment, and followed through to achieve his goal. It is important to note that he did not find it necessary to go on special diets and purchase expensive exercise equipment to accomplish his goal. This young man did choose to control his calorie intake and the quality of foods which he ate. He included walking and rock climbing as part of his physical regimen. He found some old used tires which he pulled around the yard with a strong rope. He went to the local gym for further strength building exercise. I point this out to demonstrate that anyone, including you, can achieve your goal if you truly want to! Simply learn to think and act outside the box. Stretch your imagination!

CHAPTER 15

WHAT IS THE HEART ECHO
TEST TELLING ME ?

Heart ECHO test! What a strange name for a test that measures the size, shape, and overall health of the human heart! Exactly what is it, and what does it do? More importantly, what is its function in treating heart disease?

The official name for this test is echocardiography, or diagnostic cardiac ultrasound. It uses sound waves to create pictures of your hearts chambers, valves, walls and the blood vessels (Aorta, Pulmonary Artery, veins) coming from your heart. It also carefully examines the arteries going to your heart. These are the ones that feed and nourish your heart muscle to keep it operating properly. This test is also called a heart ECHO. How does it work? A transducer, or probe as it is called, is pressed over your chest. This probe produces sound waves that bounce off your heart and "echo" back to the probe. These waves are changed into pictures viewed on a video monitor. An echo test can't harm you. There are no ill effects. The test helps your doctor find out the size and shape of your heart, and the size, thickness and movement of the walls of the heart. It shows how your heart moves and the strength of the pumping action of your heart. It also determines if the heart valves are working correctly and if blood is leaking backwards through your heart valves. (Regurgitation). The echo can also determine if the heart valves are too narrow (stenosis). If there is a tumor or infectious growth around your heart valves. Possible problems with the outer lining of your heart (the pericardium). Problems with the large blood vessels that enter and leave the heart. Blood clots in the chambers of your heart. Abnormal holes between the chambers of the heart. Remember, an echo has no risks, it cannot harm you and it does not hurt. There are no side effects. There is no reason to be alarmed if your doctor orders one for you. If ordered by your doctor, simply go. Get this done! While you're at it don't forget to thank God for one more invention by modern science to help keep you alive and well!

CHAPTER 16

EJECTION FRACTION AND SATISFACTION

One of the most important results from an echocardiogram is the ability for your doctor to measure your ejection fraction ratio. In simple layman's terms, this measures the strength and volume of the pumping action of your left ventricle which is the main pumping chamber of your heart.

Pretend you are looking at a river while standing on the bank. Perhaps you are contemplating trying your luck at fishing. There are two questions that any fisherman wants to have answered before he steps into the river. How deep is the water? How fast is the water moving? The moving river symbolizes the flow of blood throughout your body. The ejection fraction numbers measure the volume and the force of the blood as it leaves your heart.

The number 60 is the optimal number for a healthy person. After seven heart attacks, my 'EF' number is 38 which pleases me to no end! I expect it may even go higher in the next few months! Much of this is due to my newly developed lifestyle of proper eating and appropriate exercise. I believe that every day is a gift from God to be cherished and protected. Every day may be the last day of my life. I must choose to use it wisely!

CHAPTER 17

WHAT ARE THE BATHROOM SCALES TELLING ME ?

Practically every household in the United States of America has a set of bathroom scales. With this in mind there is no excuse for anyone to remain ignorant of his or her weight. Some homes have the old-fashioned spring type scales. A more modern version of the bathroom scale is equipped with batteries and a computer chip with digital readout.

Most scales don't lie! A very old scale may be off a few pounds, but this doesn't really matter. The trick is to use the same scales on a consistent basis. <u>Your most important measurement is whether you are gaining, staying the same, or losing weight.</u> Don't worry about the numbers as much as the direction in which they are moving. More money is spent, and wasted, trying to lose weight than on any other exercise. Just remember, your scales are a tool to help you reach a goal. Also remember that the goal has to be <u>your</u>

goal, no one else's. If you decide to lose weight, set yourself a reasonable goal with a reasonable timeframe to accomplish this goal. Please do not embark on a crash program or a starvation diet to achieve your goal! It's just not worth it and may do you a great deal of harm. If you choose to reduce or eliminate your intake of animal protein, refined sugar and flour, and combine this choice with a modest exercise program, you will lose weight!

A reasonable goal might be to lose one or two pounds a week. I also encourage you to weigh yourself no more than once a week. This will help eliminate the ups and downs associated with the amount of water your body maintains. Within a month or two you should know whether or not your plan is working to your satisfaction. Your scale is your friend. Your scale is your good friend. Your scale is also your private friend. No one else has a 'need to know' what your scale is telling you. This is your secret unless you wish to share. I wish you the best of luck!

CHAPTER 18

WHAT IS MY BLOOD PRESSURE TELLING ME ?

A SILENT KILLER

High blood pressure has been referred to as the silent killer of many people. High blood pressure is silent for several reasons. We cannot feel it. We cannot see it. It gives no warning signs. It is one of the killers that our body fails to warn us about. Only when our blood pressure really becomes 'high' do we begin to recognize it as something dangerous. Often this is too little, too late. What's the big deal with high blood pressure?

DANGERS OF HIGH BLOOD PRESSURE

Dangers of high blood pressure include strokes and heart attacks, and even death. It can aid in the development of killer blood clots which can break loose and travel to the heart or brain or lungs; destroying major portions of any involved organ. High blood pressure also causes the heart to work harder and adds stress to the entire circulatory system.

CAUSES OF HIGH BLOOD PRESSURE

High blood pressure is usually caused by the hardening of our arteries. When arteries lose their elasticity, the inner walls become narrowed. Which leads to diminished blood flow to our heart, brain, and every organ of our body! Stress has been shown to become a major contributing factor. Buildup of fatty plaque tissue inside the arteries further contributes to the narrowing of the inner lining of the blood vessels, raising blood pressure even more. This soon becomes an ever-increasing cycle of destruction.

NATURAL CURES

I stress once again that <u>proper diet and moderate exercise</u> can do much to lower high blood pressure to acceptable levels. There is no substitute to healthy, pliable blood vessels throughout every stage of our lives. Regular monitoring of our blood pressure is an absolute must! Household type blood pressure measuring devices are available in most drugstores without a prescription. They are relatively inexpensive. I believe it is imperative for every household to own one. It is even more important for every adult to regularly test his or her blood pressure, making lifestyle adjustments as necessary! <u>Fail to do this at your own peril!</u>

CHAPTER 19
WHAT IS THE TAPE MEASURE TELLING ME ?

Many children use a tape measure or a yardstick to measure their height while growing into adulthood. Sadly, most adults put the tape measure away when they need it most! When a gentleman shops for a pair of trousers, he needs to know two measurements. He needs to know the length of his leg and the girth of his waist. Both measurements are essential if the trousers are to fit appropriately. Some men, when becoming rather portly, seek to deny this fact by pushing their waistband lower to compensate for the bulging belly.

It goes without saying that if we continue to gain weight we will need to eventually invest in a new set of clothing. A word of caution here, the opposite is also true! I have found it necessary to trade in all of my 36-inch waist trousers for the 34-inch variety. This is a good thing!

BELLY FAT IS DANGEROUS

Dangers of excess belly fat include a higher risk of heart disease, type II diabetes and insulin resistance just to name a few. Belly fat tends to crowd many of the major organs, pushing them out of place. It's hard for an organ to do its proper job when squeezed by belly fat! Belly fat crowds your heart preventing it from squeezing out the amount of blood necessary to keep you healthy. Belly fat squeezes your lungs to add to the shortness of breath brought on by poor heart function. Belly fat makes you more inviting to a hungry bear. Belly fat also makes it more difficult for you to run away, should you encounter a hungry bear! Belly fat is almost impossible to hide. Belly fat makes you look and feel fat! Fat around your belly is the easiest type to put on and the most difficult to get rid of. However, if you stop eating animal fat, including dairy, you most certainly will start losing your belly fat! A moderate amount of exercise will hasten this process. That is my personal testimony based on my personal experience!

CHAPTER 20

WHAT ARE EMPTY PILL BOTTLES TELLING ME ?

Perhaps the most significant victory I have realized as the result of my newly found way of eating, is the fact that under the direction of my Heart Doctor I have been able to discontinue three of my prescription heart medications while reducing the amounts or strengths of several others. What a victory to realize that some are no longer needed! Those bottles are empty! All this with absolutely no negative results. All this with absolutely no signs of Angina! All this while maintaining excellent blood pressure and heart rate. I have also been able to reduce one medication for the treatment of diabetes by half, while completely eliminating another one! THIS IS MEASUREABLE PROGRESS! All because of a change to a vegetarian lifestyle!

CHAPTER 21

VICTORY EVERY DAY

ONE DAY AT A TIME

Every time that I feel tempted, I need to stop and realize that I am not alone. Satan, the sworn enemy of every Christian, wants to make us fail! If he can make you and me fail, he will succeed in making us feel guilty, which will lead to feeling depressed. Satan loves depression! After all he created it. He created depression to make us feel worthless. To make us feel unusable to God. To make us want to curl up in the fetal position and let the rest of the world go by. Let's face it folks, Satan is good at what he does. I know just how good he is. I've been there, all curled up with no place to go. Feeling like an utter failure. This gives the enemy great joy! However, God is far more powerful than Satan! God desires us to succeed! Our God is totally capable of helping us succeed. You see, God wants us to feel good about ourselves. He wants us to stand in the winner's circle. It's at that point, that He can truly use you and me for his glory. Our choice is not about winning or losing. The question is, how badly do I want to win? Do I have the courage to stay the course and win the race?

JESUS IN THE WILDERNESS

Immediately after Jesus was baptized, two things happened: "After his baptism, as Jesus came up out of the water, the heavens were opened and he saw the Spirit of God descending like a dove and settling on Him. And a voice from heaven said, this is my beloved Son and I am fully pleased with Him. Then Jesus was led out into the wilderness by the Holy Spirit to be tested there by the Devil. For forty days and forty nights he ate nothing and became very hungry. Then the Devil came and said to him, 'If you are the Son of God, change these stones into loaves of bread'. But Jesus told him, No! The Scriptures say people need more than bread for their life; they must feed on every word of God. Then the Devil took him to Jerusalem, to the highest point of the Temple, and said, if you are the Son of God, jump off! For the Scriptures say, he orders his angels to protect you and they will hold you with their hands to keep you from striking your foot on a stone. Jesus responded, the Scriptures also say do not test the Lord your God. Next the Devil took him to the peak of a very high mountain and showed him the nations of the world and all their glory. I will give it all to you he said, if you will only kneel down and worship me. Get out of here, Satan, Jesus told him. For the Scriptures say, you must worship the Lord your God; and serve Him only. Then the Devil went away and angels came and cared for Jesus" (Matthew 3:16 – 4:11).

Satan tempted Jesus because he wanted him to fail. Satan tempts you and me for the same reason. He wants us to fail. If we fail to stay healthy in our body, we will also be failing in our effort to worship God. We will be so disgusted with ourselves that we will withdraw from our Lord. Immediately following this, we will have a giant-sized load of guilt. Rest assured, guilt is a gift from the enemy. It is a special gift from Satan. I like to refer to <u>guilt</u> as '<u>the gift that keeps on giving</u>'. If Satan can load us down with guilt, he has won the victory! Let me emphasize that our victory does not happen all at once. Victory happens one day at a time. Victory can even happen one moment at a time. Every time we have victory over a temptation, it is a victory! Every time we choose to stay healthy in our body, we also are choosing to stay healthy in our spirit!

The United States of America is bordered on the west by the Pacific Ocean and on the east by the Atlantic Ocean. It is possible to walk from one ocean to the other over approximately 3,000 miles. How in the world can you do this? That's easy, just take one step at a time. Life is full of choices. We can conquer whatever difficulties we encounter as long as we face them one at a time.

CHAPTER 22

THE ISLAND OF SARDINIA

BLUE ZONES

I have recently become aware of a National Geographic researcher named Dan Buettner, author of "<u>The Blue Zones</u>", '<u>Lessons for Living Longer from the People Who've Lived the Longest</u>'. This was published in 2008 by National Geographic Partners, LLC. This book chronicles the authors' studies of the lives of Centenarians from five of the world's locations containing the greatest number of surviving, active and happy men and women over 100 years old. I am both intrigued and excited to discover the amazing correlations of their lives to many of the lessons I have shared in this book!

I first became aware of this through an article in Woman's World magazine titled "<u>Treat yourself to Longevity Soup</u>". This article starts out by introducing the Centennial population on the island of Sardinia. It then quickly moves on to state "Sardinia's longest living families still eat vegetable soup for lunch every single day." The article states how easy it is to have this tasty habit that anyone can follow using nutritious ingredients from your local supermarket. What truly made my day was the recipe which followed for their "Longevity Soup". Suffice it to say that their recipe was almost exactly the same as my vegetable soup recipe included in chapter 7 of this book! Wow!

Buettner's book covers the "Blue Zones" in Sardinia, Italy; Okinawa, Japan; Loma Linda, California; and the Nicoya Peninsula, Costa Rica. These are areas with the highest concentrations of men and women who are living and who are over 100 years of age. I have chosen to limit my observations here to the 100 + year old men in the small mountain village of Barbagia, in Sardinia, Italy. These Centenarian men were hard working shepherds or farmers who had worked hard all of their lives. Most of them had worked well into their 80's or more. They typically walked three to five miles daily over mountainous terrains to herd their sheep or tend to their crops. Most importantly, their diets had consistently been made up of fresh vegetables, whole grain bread, and modest amounts of red wine. They ate very little meat and almost no fish. They lived with extended family and shared family duties. Many were known to laugh loudly and often. They enjoyed their simple lifestyle and the beauty of their surroundings. The Centenarians in this village were found to be very similar to most of the Centenarians he interviewed in each of the four "Blue Zones" covered in this excellent book.

I found myself mesmerized by this book. Mr. Buettner emphasized three factors that were found among Centenarians throughout the regions he studied. These folks had a sense of purpose for their lives combined with a sense of humor. They had strong family ties and support with genuine love displayed. Finally, they all had a healthy lifestyle including hard work and healthy, vegetarian style diets.

After reading this book and reflecting on the findings, I find myself rejoicing in the fact that my observations concerning heart health also have a much greater scope for living a healthy, long, and fulfilling life. Who knows? You and I may well be able to extend the quality as well as the longevity of our lives by changing how we live and how we eat! I am truly grateful to Mr. Buettner for his most informative study. We may live to be 100 years old after all!

CHAPTER 23

LIVING AND SHARING THE GOOD NEWS

Most decisions in life have both a positive and a negative consequence. The trickiest part of making decisions comes when we need to weigh one side against the other. What will I lose, what will I gain?

So, I ask the question, "Are you ready to make the commitment to change your eating habits for the rest of your life"? Weigh your commitment carefully before you answer. Your positive commitment will not only change your quality of life but may also add years to your life!

I, BILL YEOMANS, HAVE MADE THE DECISION
AND THE COMMITMENT TO CHANGE THE
WAY I EAT
AND TO CONTROLWHAT I EAT
IN ORDER TO PROMOTE MY OWN QUALITY
OF LIFE

AND TO EXTEND MY LENGTH OF LIFE
TO SERVE MY CREATOR AND MY LORD.

WITH THAT AS MY FOCUS,
I PRESENT THIS BOOK TO YOU.
THIS IS MY TESTIMONY TO YOU
AND MY PRAYER FOR YOU.

CHAPTER 24

KEEP YOUR BLESSINGS FLOWING

"It is more blessed to give than to receive" (Acts 20:35). There was a popular Christian song around 1960 titled "Pass it on". One of the verses states that "It only takes a spark to get a fire going... So, it is with God's love, once you've experienced it..." The essence of that song is that you cannot keep God's love only for yourself. It is imperative that we pass it on to a world that desperately needs to be reconciled to God.

God is calling every Christian to be a messenger of truth, a messenger of love, and a messenger of personal victory through Jesus Christ our Lord. Will you answer His call?

INDEX

Further Resources for Your Consideration

The China Study © 2006 by T. Colin Campbell, Ph.D., and Thomas M. Campbell II
First Bella Books, Dallas, Texas

Prevent and Reverse Heart Disease ©2007 by Caldwell B. Essleton Jr., M.D.
The Penguin Group, New York, NY 10014

Dr. Dean Ornish's Program for Reversing Heart Disease ©2010 by Dean Ornish
Ivy Books, publisher, New York, NY

Dr. Neal Barnard's Program for Reversing Diabetes © 2007 by Neal D. Barnard, M.D.
Rodale, Inc. New York, NY 10017

The End of Diabetes © 2013 by Joel Fuhrman, M.D.
HarperCollins, New York, NY 10022

Eat to Live © 2003 by Joel Fuhrman, M.D.
Little, Brown and company, New York, New York

The Whole Heart Solution © 2013 Joel K. Kahn, M.D.
The Reader's Digest Association, Inc., White Plains, NY 10601

The Senior's Guide to Metabolism ©2011 by FC&A
Publishing,
Peachtree City, GA 30269

Eat More, Weigh Less ©1993 by Dean Ornish
HarperCollins Publishers, Inc., New York, NY 10022

What Your doctor may Not Tell You About Heart Disease
©2012 by Mark Houston, M.D.

Grand Central Life and Style   Hatchette Book Group, New
York, NY 10017

The Nitric Oxide Solution ©2010 Neogenis, Austin, TX
78746 by Nathan S. Bryan, Ph.D. and Janet Zand, OMD

NO More Heart Disease ©2005 by Healthwell Ventures
St. Martin's Press, New York, NY 10010 by Louis J. Ignarro

The Blue Zones ©2008 by Dan Buettner
National Geographic Partners, LLC

BOOKS BY THIS AUTHOR

Book 1   <u>Power Versus</u> – To Strengthen Your Walk

Book 2   <u>The Face of God</u> – Reflected in Nature

A Three Book Volume: 'Things that Matter'

Book 3   <u>Christ Centered Marriages</u> – Your Marriage Matters, Vol. 1

Book 4   <u>Christ Centered Finances</u> – Your Money Matters, Vol. 2

Book 5   <u>Christ Centered Families</u> – Your Kids Matter, Vol. 3

Book 6   <u>Bill I AM</u> – An Autobiography

Book 7   <u>My Heart MADE NEW</u>

Each of these titles is available on AMAZON and also on Kindle E-Books

IN THE PIPELINE

Book 8   The Spirit of God

Book 9   America Needs God

BOOK 10   Tough Men for Tough Times